Overcoming Panic and Related Anxiety Disorders

Margaret Hawkins began her career as a junior library assistant. This gave her a passion for books, but it was not until she became ill with anxiety problems that she started to write herself. Unable to find simple and sound explanations for what was becoming a living nightmare, she found that – except for material written by 'experts' containing much medical data – there was little help. Her work for the charity No Panic has provided a wonderful opportunity to research and strengthen her ideas on methods of recovery from all types of anxiety disorders. This book is the consequence of that work and experience.

Overcoming Common Problems Series

Selected titles

A full list of titles is available from Sheldon Press,
36 Causton Street, London SW1P 4ST and on our website at
www.sheldonpress.co.uk

Overcoming Common Problems

Overcoming Panic and Related Anxiety Disorders

MARGARET HAWKINS

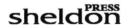
sheldon PRESS

Grateful thanks to Peter, my husband,
for his patience and stoicism

First published in Great Britain in 2009

Sheldon Press
36 Causton Street
London SW1P 4ST

British Library Cataloguing-in-Publication Data
A catalogue record for this book is available from the British Library

ISBN 978-1-84709-061-4

1 3 5 7 9 10 8 6 4 2

Typeset by Fakenham Photosetting Ltd, Fakenham, Norfolk
Printed in Great Britain by Ashford Colour Press

Produced on paper from sustainable forests

Essex County
Council Libraries

Contents

Acknowledgements

I would like to thank Colin M. Hammond MBE, founder of No Panic, for his support; Kevin Gournay CBE, Professor Emeritus at the Institute of Psychiatry, for his willingness to help and answer my questions, and Jeremy Dyson, writer and actor, who read my previous work and gave me the encouragement I needed to continue writing. Finally, my thanks go to Fiona Marshall at Sheldon Press, who has been a tower of strength.

Introduction

Am I ill in the accepted sense? No, I'm not. I don't conform. I haven't got a virus, no broken bones, my heart and lungs are functioning well, so my doctor tells me. What is the matter then? If I'm not ill, why do I feel ill and sometimes look ill? I have all the pre-requisites – pains in my chest, breathing problems, can't eat because my throat seems to close, can't walk because my legs are like jelly, and then there are the dizzy spells. I've got to be ill, haven't I?

Let me think again. These are all real symptoms that I am experiencing, but just supposing I accepted that I was not physically ill, what would I be left with – just that, a collection of symptoms. But why do I have them?

I've been told that it is because I am anxious and that the strange feelings are produced by my nervous system, which is not as steady as it should be. Apparently, surges of adrenaline are causing these frightening things to happen to me. Yet, I don't ask for them to happen, so why do they?

I can't remember exactly when it started. It may have been when I lost my job, or was it when the baby was born and I was so stressed? Perhaps it was when I had to move to another area and I was lonely, or was it after Dad died? Maybe it was the time when I had to have that operation or perhaps it was the divorce. I don't know!

So, here I am with a cluster of symptoms that I can't get rid of because I don't know what to do. Let me think about this. The first panic attack I had occurred in the street. It was unexpected and a tremendous shock. Of course it could have happened anywhere, when I was held up in traffic, at the shops, in the office or even at home. When I look back, I can see that because I was so scared of the horrible feelings, I soon started to avoid the places and situations that made me anxious. However, before all this occurred I had no problem with these situations. So, what does that tell me?

I've been reassured that I am physically well, but something must trigger off these attacks. What can it be? I've tried to ignore them. I've kept away from distressing situations. I've tried everything, but nothing seems to work. On the whole I don't feel too bad as long as I don't rock the boat, but I *want* to rock the boat. I want to do all the things I used to do.

It appears that only my thoughts are left. It must be something to do with them. They say that the mind is like a computer, so I suppose what I have done is save my experiences as a personal document. Consequently, when I am having a bad day I automatically search through my memory bank and pull out the file that reads, 'You felt frightened when you were in this situation before.' That is quite enough to make me feel frightened all over again! Unfortunately, I have put the wrong information into my 'computer' and have consciously or unconsciously created an invalid program. What am I going to do? Well, I am going to rewrite my program so that when I do a search the new document will now read, 'I know I felt frightened in this situation before, but I must remember that I haven't always reacted like this. The situation has not changed, just my conception of it. I am afraid of a feeling that I had, and now I'm recreating it.'

My computer can only do what I tell it and it has to follow the program through. In other words, if I think 'I might panic' my inbuilt computer starts to search its memory bank to locate all the things connected with this thought and it sends out messages, alarm signals, that work automatically to get me ready for action. But, I don't need to go into action – there is nothing for me to fight! I am going to try and accept what has happened to me and gradually go through my memory file deleting all the old and unwanted information. After that, I am going to write a new program that will give me a different perspective on my problems and finally banish fear.

My experience

One evening in June, some years ago I was walking home alone, when to my puzzlement I noticed that the road seemed to be undulating. It appeared to be heaving like the waves of the sea. I stopped still and then saw that the garden walls were leaning towards me. I began to feel rather scared and my heart started to beat rapidly. I tried to walk forward but my vision was becoming blurred to such an extent that the only object I could register was a fluorescent light on a distant building. By now I was terrified and my one thought was that I must get home. I recognized the light: it was from a hotel not far from where I lived. I concentrated on this and ran frantically towards it. Eventually I got home. My husband greeted me and I blurted out that I must be ill. He was shocked. There was a thumping beat in my head and I couldn't breathe properly.

The doctor came and examined me, looking for a reason to explain what had occurred. After some considerable time he said that he could not find anything physically wrong that would have caused the problem. 'It must be your nerves,' he said. I was astounded and replied, 'But I have never suffered from "nerves" and have never been a nervous person.' At this point he suggested that I should not venture out for a few days and that he would give me some pills for my 'nerves'.

In retrospect, there was an obvious pattern emerging from my childhood experiences, but I did not register this at the time. I was so happy and secure that it seemed unimaginable that I could even be considered as a nervous individual. I lived life to the full. Why had this happened to me? Apparently it had come out of the blue, from nowhere, uncultivated and alien to my personality. The years that followed became a journey of discovery, questioning the reasons for panic and anxiety disorders. When I was plunged unceremoniously into the deep, dark pit of panic it was at a time when little was known about such a thing by general practitioners, even less by the general public and my own ignorance was total. It took me ten years of self-education to sort out the intricacies of how thoughts and feelings played a major part in keeping me in my cage of anxiety. It was extremely difficult, but I had to persevere for the sake of my family as well as myself. Thankfully, for you who may be reading this, understanding of anxiety disorders has moved forwards in leaps and bounds, and nowadays no one should have to suffer from these terrible illnesses without help. There is a way through and I am going to provide you with the tools.

How did I cope? What did I do? First, I knew that at all costs I must try to go out. I managed to do this by asking a friend if she would accompany me, as the thought of being 'out there' alone was too much to bear. I walked out with my friend and my dog every day; sometimes I felt panicky, but I soldiered on through the feelings regardless, even though I was exhausted by the effort. It was a great day when we went to town on the bus. I went on family holidays too, but panic was there with me and life was a constant battle.

At some point I decided that I would avidly read everything I could find about anxiety disorders. I learnt that the body could become sensitized. This led me to work on muscle relaxation and also how to breathe, slowly and evenly, from the diaphragm, to counteract the feelings caused by rushes of adrenaline. I intend to share with you in this book all the information and experience that I have gathered. Today I am a different being and, though a predisposition to panic may always remain, 'it' and I have come to a comfortable arrangement, I live calmly and 'it' doesn't visit me any more.

For the last 15 years I have worked with the National Organization for Phobias, Anxiety Neuroses, Information and Care (No Panic). I originally trained to work on the Helpline and then took further training to enable me to train others for Helpline work. I graduated to take Recovery Groups, train Recovery Group Leaders and take charge of publicity for the charity. I have for the last two years had the privilege of being the elected Chairperson. I have met some extraordinary people who have lived in constant terror but, through understanding that they could take charge of their illness, have come through the misery of panic, agoraphobia and other related anxiety illnesses and are now able to function without fear.

Note: This is not a medical book and is not intended to replace advice from your doctor. Do consult your doctor if you are experiencing symptoms with which you feel you need help.

1

Why panic?

What causes our first panic attack? Why do we get that sudden surge of adrenaline that consumes and terrifies us and appears to come 'out of the blue'? Several reasons may come to mind but they usually do so with the benefit of hindsight. We may have a predisposition to anxiety, which together with a build-up of stressful life experiences, has brought us to this precise moment. Sometimes we can discover what has happened to make us so vulnerable, but knowing does not mean that we will become well instantly. Our bodies and minds have to readjust and we have much to learn about how to bring this change about.

James for instance had been the carer of his parents for 15 years. His father died and then, six months later, his mother died too. James felt totally isolated. He had no close friends as he had not been in a position to cultivate relationships, and he had now become frightened of being alone. Nights were the worst. His pattern of sleep was erratic; he would wake suddenly, bathed in perspiration as panic engulfed him. To combat his terror and to hear a friendly human voice he spent the early hours of the morning calling radio stations that invited people to ring them. Having been under such physical and mental pressure for such a long time it was not surprising that James began to experience panic. His life had been turned upside down and he had lost his purpose and his motivation.

Lily, though married, was a career girl at heart and had made great progress in her job. Now she had a baby to care for and, though she loved the child dearly, she found herself resenting the fact that she was unable to work. One day she felt dizzy and faint. She ignored this episode as it passed quite quickly. She continued doing everything for the baby and struggling to keep her home clean and welcoming. She became more and more tired but brushed her feelings aside until one day when she was in the garden, hanging washing on the clothes line, she began to feel uneasy, not quite sure of what was happening. All around her looked blurred and hazy but the sound of the birds singing

1

seemed heightened. Lily started to breathe rapidly and she felt a rush of adrenaline course through her body, she dropped the clothes basket and ran indoors terrified.

After suffering more panic attacks Lily went to see her doctor who discovered that she was anaemic; this had caused Lily to become very debilitated and had contributed to her becoming anxious.

It is not unusual to be unaware that for a period of time we may have been living with a high anxiety level, and eventually there comes a point when our body cannot cope and it rebels. The surge of adrenaline is inappropriate at that time. We don't need it. Adrenaline is energy expending, for example when we are exercising, so when panic appears to come from 'out of the blue' – perhaps when we are sitting watching television or out shopping – is it any wonder that we are shaken and afraid? Not only that, but just look at the symptoms that anxiety and panic can produce! Pains in the chest, breathing problems, inability to swallow, legs that feel like jelly and dizziness – to name but a few. Of course, it is only natural that we want to avoid those nasty feelings and the horrible experience we have been through and that's where we make our first mistake.

Avoidance is disaster. If we could only believe that a panic attack is just adrenaline accompanied by a collection of symptoms that cannot and will not harm us, we'd soon improve. Unfortunately, because we are so afraid, our thinking plays a major part in sustaining that terror. The 'what if' syndrome comes into play: 'What if it comes again? What if I faint? What if I can't get home, get help?' The mindless questions go on and on as we torment ourselves.

So, the first panic occurs for a reason that we may, or may not be able to establish positively, the second and subsequent panic attacks do not. As US sportsman Jerry Augustine once said, 'The body manifests what the mind harbours.' That's worth remembering.

Hyperventilation

You may be aware that breathing can have a role in how you feel, but possibly you haven't fully recognized how fast, shallow breathing, or hyperventilation, affects the development of a full-blown panic attack.

So, what is hyperventilation? What does it do? What can we do to remedy the problem? I am hoping that I can shed a little more light on this common but sometimes frightening symptom. What is it? Basically it is breathing inappropriately. When you run up stairs, you are not in the least surprised when your breathing becomes rapid. You know that it will slow down and adjust automatically. Normally, you don't think about your breathing – it just happens naturally – but when you are not doing anything to cause you to breathe more quickly, for instance, if you are just sitting watching television and you become aware that this is happening, it is not appropriate.

What does this mean? Breathing inappropriately can cause very unpleasant feelings because an imbalance is occurring in the bloodstream, so that the balance of oxygen and carbon dioxide is disturbed. Air taken in through the nose or mouth travels through the bloodstream, where tissues take up the oxygen that they need. They then throw out the carbon dioxide as rubbish, back into the bloodstream, through the lungs and out through the nose or mouth. The body always retains sufficient oxygen, which it carries around via its red blood cells that are usually 98–99 per cent full of oxygen. Therefore, however much over-breathing you do, you cannot overload your blood with more oxygen than is necessary.

The more important factor is the carbon dioxide. When you over-breathe you lose too much carbon dioxide. In the base of the brain, there is a control mechanism which measures the levels of carbon dioxide in the blood and decides what to do to keep our breathing balanced. It sends messages to the body as to how we should be breathing. If you habitually breathe quickly and have done so for some time, the control mechanism will adjust to a lower level, but unfortunately does not give much room for manoeuvre. You are close to triggering off your problem, and just one more big breath – even a big sigh or yawn – can be enough to throw out the last little bit of carbon dioxide, unbalancing your breathing sufficiently to cast you into a spiral of symptoms. It is very similar to the part that adrenaline plays in producing panic. If anxiety and stress become a habit, the body becomes sensitized and is triggered more easily into panic.

In hyperventilation, when the breathing control centre in the brain adjusts to a lower level, this is when the feelings of light-headedness, pins and needles, and a feeling of being unable to catch a breath occur. There are other symptoms too, such as chilled hands and feet, unreality, visual problems, difficulty in swallowing, muscle pains, cramps and many more. Strangely, people who are hyperventilating constantly may not appear to be particularly short of breath, as they do not seem to be gasping or panting rapidly – their bodies have become used to breathing this way. Again, compare this with someone having a panic attack; do you notice anything particularly extraordinary in his or her behaviour? You could be standing next to someone, and may not even be aware that this is happening.

What can we do to remedy the situation?

We have to retrain our breathing and get our breathing control centre to readjust and climb back to its correct level. The aim is to start to take control of our breathing by slowing it down. This is achieved by gradually learning how to breathe in an even, constant rhythm, filling the lungs completely by using the diaphragmatic muscle, keeping the upper chest as still as possible. At first you may not be able to manage to slow your breathing down very much but the more you practise the more adept you will become, gradually reducing the amount of breaths you take in per minute.

Don't take too deep a breath and don't force the air out – control is what we want to achieve. Breathe in through the nose, and also out through the nose. There is a reason for doing this. If you breathe in through the mouth, cold air entering the back of the throat can make you feel as if you need to take another breath quickly. Breathing correctly through the nose means that you are taking clean air into the lungs, air that is warm and moist, filtered by the hairs in the nose. Air taken in through the mouth is not only cold and dry but dirtier too. An anxious person who breathes out through the mouth is more likely to breathe in through the mouth simply because he or she is not yet able to control his or her breathing. It is likely that someone who is unsure will, after breathing out through the mouth, feel the need to take an extra breath. When this happens, the person tends to take the next breath in through the mouth, and this can sometimes make one gulp or yawn, thus exacerbating the problem. So, it is important to concentrate, and to inhale and exhale through the nose.

However, at some point, as you are learning to slow down your breathing, you may indeed feel that you simply have to take a bigger breath. This happens because you are actually achieving something – you are raising the carbon dioxide level in your blood, and your control centre is telling you to get rid of it by breathing more. Here, again, we can compare it to the feeling one gets when learning to relax, the feeling of uncertainty, slight panic even, because your body is not used to feeling this way and is trying to readjust. When learning to breathe correctly the same sort of thing may occur. Don't be afraid of this. It is very important, as it means that you are beginning to raise the carbon dioxide level in your blood, making the control centre return to its proper level. If you do feel overwhelmed, you can take a bigger breath but it must be through the nose and controlled by the diaphragm, breathing gently, slowly and evenly, and this will reduce the sensation. It takes courage, determination and practice but it *is* possible to take control of your breathing if you really want to.

2

What really happens in a panic attack – and why it can't hurt you

Ten thousand years ago Lugg and his partner Penna were walking through the forest looking for berries. Penna said, 'Lugg, are you sure there aren't any tigers in this forest?' Lugg laughed and said, 'No! The tribe has killed them all. Don't worry!' But Penna felt a bit anxious, especially as the forest was getting thicker and darker. Suddenly there was a strange noise and the two humans froze in their tracks. Their hearts thumped violently. Lugg reached for his long spear while Penna picked up a sharp rock. They tiptoed cautiously along the path until Penna glimpsed a flash of colour to their right. Instantly she hurled the rock at it and together she and Lugg charged towards it screaming as loudly as they could. But it wasn't a tiger after all. Lugg laughed with relief. 'Look,' he said, 'it's only a squirrel. I told you not to worry!'

When someone is depleted physically and mentally, the nervous system plays a major part in their illness. The way they think causes automatic responses from the nervous system, which is out of kilter, sensitized, and ready to spring into action if it gets signals that indicate danger may be imminent. A simple way of describing how this works is to imagine that the brain is shaped like a circle. (I do know that the brain is not really shaped like a circle, but I'm trying to convey my ideas in the easiest way possible!) So, to continue, mentally draw a horizontal line through the centre of the circle. One half of the circle now represents the thinking part of the brain, and the other half the nervous system. Then divide the nervous system (the bottom half, see Fig. 2.1) in half vertically so that it is in two sections. These two sections represent the sympathetic and parasympathetic branches of the Automatic Nervous or Autonomic Nervous System, as it is sometimes called.

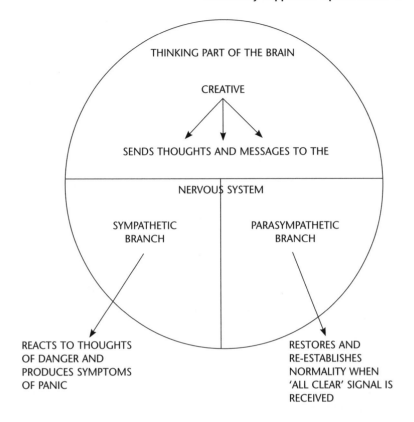

Figure 2.1: Simplified working of the brain and nervous system

The thinking part of the brain is creative and cannot actually do anything to prepare us physically. Conversely, the automatic nervous system can perform routine tasks but it cannot think or rationalize. Everything it does is programmed. It supervises our heartbeat, the way our lungs inflate and deflate, it takes care of our digestive system, in fact all the functions that keep us alive. Without it, we would have to remember to breathe, pump our heart, etc., and if you have a memory like mine I don't think we would survive for very long!

Anxiety symptoms are not intangible. They become a learned process and response. Our inbuilt computer does not make an error; it is we who program it and put in the wrong information that cause the fault. The next step is logical too. We have to challenge and re-program our thinking patterns so that we do not give the wrong commands to our nervous system, which has no choice but to react automatically.

The nervous system is triggered by the senses, seeing, hearing, taste, touch and smell. We are using these senses constantly, so why does the nervous system get triggered sometimes and not others? It is because of memory. If we have a frightening experience that causes us to panic, this gets stored away in our mind and at a later date one of our senses picks up a trigger that reminds us of that scary situation. In other words, we store away the horrible feelings we had when we experienced our first panic attack and so our nervous system starts to get our body ready for running away or standing to fight.

These are primitive instincts that are necessary in a dangerous situation but not useful when we are not in any kind of peril. Remember Lugg and Penna in the forest? They had a real reason to worry; they could have been attacked by a tiger. We are not in such a situation – the worst thing that could happen is a quite specific, repetitive set of symptoms. The symptoms you produce with your first panic attack will probably not alter very much and may well be exactly the same if you have further attacks. Other people may have different feelings but you cannot 'catch' them or create identical ones; what you feel depends on your personal body make-up. So if you meet someone who has different symptoms from yours, don't start thinking that you might get them too, because you won't.

Why does this preparation take place when we are not in danger? The answer lies in the level of anxiety. If it is too high and has remained high for a period of time, the body becomes sensitized. It's rather like looking at a barbecue where the charcoal appears grey, ashy and dead but you only have to give the coals one little poke and they will burst into flames. All the heat is underneath – similar to the anxiety, which is sustaining a constantly high level ready for action. If we were in an upsetting situation previously and we panicked, now our memory connects with that situation and our senses trigger off the automatic reaction. For instance, suppose we had been trapped in a lift and couldn't get out, isn't it logical that the feelings that were aroused on that occasion are recreated when we find ourselves stuck, say, in a traffic jam? Confusion reigns as each part of our nervous system tries to do its job. To all intents and purposes there is no direct way that the brain can stop the spiral of panic – the adrenaline rush – once it has started. This is the crux of the problem. The thinking part of our brain may shout, 'STOP' but it won't have any effect because it has no physical input, unlike the nervous system, which is just the opposite and has input but cannot think for itself at all. So that's the problem we have to overcome. There we are, perhaps starting to panic, and whatever we think or say to ourselves won't have any real effect. Everything follows automatically. Each branch of the nervous system is trying to do its job and we end up with a seesaw effect. To control the nervous system we have to challenge it physically.

Imagine standing outside a pair of heavy swing doors and someone pushes through and lets them go. You can see that the doors are swinging back towards you and you can't move out of the way because other people have filled the space behind you. It's quite obvious that you are going to be knocked down. What do you do? Naturally your brain is working overtime and you are aware of what is going to happen but you cannot say to the doors, 'Stop, you are going to hurt me!' Even if you did, it wouldn't have any effect. You will either jump to one side or put out your hands to catch the doors as they come towards you.

Now can you see what I am getting at? To control the automatic nervous system and to stop the upward spiral of panic it has to be challenged physically. We can do this by learning breathing and relaxation techniques. These techniques help to control the symptoms of anxiety – those symptoms of which we are so afraid because we think that they come from an outside source, when the reality is just the opposite. Anxiety symptoms seen in these terms are a natural bodily response. They are not intangible. They form part of a learned thought process – so we need to challenge our thinking patterns and reprogram our inbuilt computer in order not to give the wrong commands to our nervous system.

Let's try and get things into some sort of perspective. What are we afraid of? The basis of our worry is the fear of fear. What holds us back when we know the fear is irrational? This is the reality, the fact, but how do we cope even though we know this to be the case? We are still at a loss.

So what *can* we do? Well, there are several things. Primarily we need to relax and release the tension that has built up in our muscles. Doing muscle relaxation daily will bring down the level of anxiety, so desensitizing our body. This means that it will not be triggered so easily, allowing us time to work on our uneasiness by breathing from the diaphragm, slowly and evenly until the pre-panic feelings subside. We need not experience panic constantly.

Changing our lifestyle, too, can be beneficial if it is not helping our situation, and a reasonable diet that keeps our blood sugar at a constant level may also help. I will talk more about this later in the book.

Are you a dweller or seeker?

Dorothy was a dweller. She sat at home and considered her problem and after much heart-searching decided that she was far too ill to go out at all. Each day she would look through her window and watch the world go by, but she felt that she was different from those people who appeared to have not a care. If they felt like her then they would not be able to stride off without worrying. Dorothy did her shopping through catalogues and spent long hours choosing her clothes and household goods. She was becoming quite a hoarder but she believed that she was entitled to spend because it was her only pleasure. Any attempt by her family to encourage her to go outside was rejected vehemently. Didn't they know how poorly she was? She was the one suffering from this terrible anxiety.

Harry was a seeker. He was intelligent – a workaholic in fact – and then he had a panic attack. He was devastated. How could this possibly have happened to him? He decided that he would get the best help available, no matter where he had to go or how much it would cost. During the following months, he travelled to see psychologists, psychiatrists, in fact anyone who would listen. He had hypnotherapy, took various pills and potions, underwent any and every kind of therapy on offer, but he didn't get better; in fact, he got worse. His panic attacks were more frequent than ever. What he didn't comprehend was that no one could make him well; he was the only person who could achieve that. It was his turn to listen to himself and with the assistance of others begin the journey of recovery.

How do you view yourself? Are you the kind of person who wants to go out into the wide world and seek adventure? Maybe you are the type of person who loves to be at home, and the thought of strange places does not appeal at all. Are there only the two options in life? No, of course not, but due to our anxieties we tend to fall into one or the other of these categories. How does this affect your anxiety illness? Perhaps you are desperately seeking a cure, restless and exhausted. Or maybe you are relieved that because you have an anxiety illness you can use it as an excuse not to step forward into the unknown. We are all so different. However, to fulfil our true potential, is it not sensible to look at both sides of the argument?

Take the home dwellers, those who appear to be quite content to stay within their safety zone. What are they missing? Enormous opportunities to see new horizons and beautiful vistas, make new friends, enjoy new experiences and acquire new skills that will allow their minds to grow instead of stagnating. Physically and mentally, without some expansion, they are existing not living.

What about the seekers though, who cannot be content but are constantly alert to their symptoms and who want to be 'normal' right now. Not in a week's time, a month or a year, but right now. They force themselves forward recklessly. Their insistent cry for cure is exhausting and their minds are overwrought with the continual search for answers to their problems. They have no time for deep thought or contemplation; they are too agitated to think logically.

Have you decided what you are: a seeker or a dweller? Can we not learn from each other? It's never too late to learn to look at things from a different perspective and it's never too late to try out different ways of doing things.

If you are a seeker, take a portion of the dweller's seeming contentment and slow down. Create a calmness through relaxation to enable yourself to realize that one cannot live satisfactorily and happily on a roller coaster. Why increase your anxiety with doses of adrenaline daily by over-reacting to your symptoms? You are not in a race; stop, look around you, smell the flowers, bask in the sunshine and just 'be' in the present. Your body will thank you and your constant introspection will ease.

If you are a dweller, sitting at home pretending that all is well, isn't it time to venture forth? Take a little piece of the seeker's energy and decide that you can make an effort towards something specific. Important occasions, family festivities – do you really want to miss them all? No, of course you don't, but sitting at home, thinking only and not making some physical attempt, will never create enough motivation. You are tired, too, I know, but exercising your body will bring a different feeling and invigorate your senses enabling you to go forward and grasp your dreams.

The role of fear in nervous illnesses

Sometimes people have suffered from a nervous episode, maybe in their youth or later on in life, and have, as they put it, 'been ill ever since'; never recovered. It is as if they have put this nervous episode into a glass jar and preserved it. Metaphorically, they carry it with them everywhere, even though it is awkward and a nuisance, but they feel that they have to keep it close so that they can watch what it is doing. On good days they can forget it for a while, though they seem to find it necessary to unscrew the lid and check to make sure it is still there. They will look at it, taste and smell the aroma of fear, touch it to see if there is any response. They may even try talking it into submission, though there is an unfortunate tendency to listen to its suggestions, and the aftermath is fairly predictable – a nervous reaction of varying degrees.

The illness will never be conquered if it is constantly being monitored to see if it is getting worse, turning mouldy like a pot of jam. The pot of jam is not subjected to scrutiny every time the cupboard door is opened. The lid is not removed and the contents tasted. Why is that? It's because we trust the ingredients and know that they have gone through a series of processes that make them edible and acceptable.

To preserve anything at all it has to be dealt with appropriately, whether it is a painting or a pot of jam. If the right techniques or additives are not used then the painting or the pot of jam will gradually deteriorate. Therefore doesn't it make sense to apply similar methods to nervous illnesses? What techniques do we need? What methods shall we include in our recipe for recovery?

Nervous illnesses are perpetuated by the misunderstanding and misuse of the senses. We recreate anxiety symptoms by thought and memory. If we change our thought patterns to positive thinking, practise diaphragmatic breathing, use muscle relaxation daily and eat a sensible diet, then we have all the right ingredients, the right techniques. Mix them to a smooth consistency and you have a good chance of recovery. All those negative thoughts you have been preserving carefully for years and years have been fermenting, changing the way you think; now may be the time to challenge their validity. Perhaps you had a very bad experience a long time ago and it made you so frightened that panic was the result. Have you had that same devastating experience again in the intervening days, months or years? I doubt it. You may have had frightening moments, panic even, but I can guarantee that those moments were in some way a result of your thinking processes.

It's not easy to venture from your comfort zone. I know that the way you cope with your life is to retreat from the situations that you think will make you ill. Coping with your fears this way makes it impossible to know what would have happened if you'd faced your demons. What is the most extreme scenario that could result from trying? You won't fade away. At the very worst you might hyperventilate or panic but you have experienced those feelings before and survived. If you have put your efforts into getting the recovery techniques correct and balanced then the possibility of hyperventilating or panicking is zero. Your mind and body are working together as one unit. You are no longer fooling your nervous system by giving it false information that makes it respond to a situation that is not life threatening.

It sounds easy, doesn't it? Yet of course it's not. Time has elapsed and habits have been formed, both mentally and physically. These habits may feel as if they are set in concrete and impossible to break down but they are only superficial really. A consistent attack will demolish them, and you will be free from the chains of terror, able to do what you want, when you want. Isn't it worth a try?

3

Feelings of unreality – high anxiety and anger

High anxiety

The worry of 'going mad'

Do you feel sometimes that the world is going on around you and that you are not part of it? When you are in a crowd do you feel isolated and unable to make connections with other people? Have you ever felt that you don't know who you are? Or where you are, even though you are on familiar ground? Do you feel 'spaced out' as if you don't know what to do next or where to go to be safe? If so, it's not surprising that you feel scared and think you must be on the verge of going mad. Hopefully I can help to dissipate this worry by telling you about the difference between psychosis and neurosis.

A neurosis is a concern of the nervous system. It involves the senses: sight, touch, taste, hearing and smell. Therefore, whatever we see, touch, taste, hear or smell that in some way frightens us, the sensory nerves send messages of warning to the brain, this then triggers the nervous system into action to help protect us. A nervous person has insight. She knows she has a problem. The psychotic person, on the other hand, may have no insight. He may not understand that something is wrong and his contact with the outside world is impaired.

Have you ever sat outside in the sunshine and then gone indoors and noticed that it takes quite a few moments for your eyes to focus properly? This is a normal occurrence and you accept it. When your anxiety is at a high level your senses become heightened and your responses rapid. That is why perhaps when we go into a supermarket and are met by noise, bright lights and bustle our anxiety level shoots up immediately, but unnecessarily. When you understand why your anxiety has been triggered and that the way to deal with it is to slow down your breathing, then it will all fall into perspective.

I have found, too, that if you move out of the situation that you are in when this occurs, it will bring you back to reality. I don't mean run away from it but 'change your position' in some way. For instance, if you are in a crowd and feel unreal, then do something positive to bring you back to the 'here and now'. It may be speaking to someone or doing something physical. It is difficult to make specific suggestions without knowing where you are or what you may be doing when you get these feelings but I can recall, for example, once feeling very anxious while out driving in the country. I stopped the car and got out, leaned on a five-barred gate, felt the breeze on my face and came back to reality very quickly. This is what I am trying to convey when I say 'change your position'. Don't sit or stand there suffering, do something! Finally, the less mindful attention you pay to unreality, the quicker it will be extinguished through lack of mental nourishment.

Why did this happen to me?

How did you come to be like this? Probably combinations of different stressful occurrences and situations have brought you to this point. However, it serves no real purpose, if one is unaware of what created the problem, to struggle to find the answer, as this will be unlikely to effect a cure. We have to deal with where we are at today. The past has gone for ever and we cannot alter it in any way, shape or form. So don't waste time and effort looking backwards.

Imagine yourself on a journey, walking with a haversack over your shoulders and carrying a bag in each hand. During this journey of life, along the way you pick up certain things and put them into your bags – for example, illness, abuse, jealousy, low self-esteem – and each of these represents a large rock. As you walk on, the bags get heavier and heavier but still you add more weight in varying degrees, remorse perhaps or anger, worry, family commitments, guilt, inadequacy, bad habits. You keep putting more and more stones into your bags that are bulging so much that, by now, you can barely lift them. Your body begins to rebel. It says, 'I can't cope with this.'

Your head aches, your shoulders are hunched up around your ears; your back feels as if it will break with the effort of trying to carry all this excess baggage. Then it gets worse, your legs start to tremble, your heart is pounding and the perspiration starts to trickle. You feel sick and dizzy and your eyes may be playing tricks on you. Finally, your body says, 'That's it, I've had enough.' The inevitable follows – a massive rush of adrenaline, and what is the result? Your first panic attack.

Basically, what I am saying is that your body has been living with anxiety and tension for some time and understandably there comes a crisis point. Your nervous system is adrift and this brings you to the situation that you find yourself in today, of being so terrified. But what are we really afraid of? We are afraid of having another attack. Why is that? Because we are afraid of the feelings of fear. We are terrified of what might happen next. We don't know what it will be but we are sure that it will be horrendous. We are constantly on the alert. This is how we fuel our anxiety. It can be triggered by a conversation, something we read in the newspaper or see on TV. Even a fleeting thought, passing through our mind so quickly that we hardly register it, can produce an automatic reaction.

Having suffered our first panic attack we tend to narrow our horizons because of the 'what if?' factor: 'I can't go shopping; I dare not take a job, because what if it happens again?' Our minds and bodies become so tired of battling with our fears. Think of the barbecue again – the coals can look grey as if the fire has gone out, but just give the ashes a little poke and the flames will appear again. This is exactly what we are like. It only needs a little prod to start us spinning off into another attack.

What can we do about it? Well, I am going to tell you how to make a start by learning how to use breathing and relaxation techniques to counteract our bodily symptoms and, later, how to use cognitive therapy to change our 'What ifs' into 'So whats'.

Pinball panic

I was thinking of how to describe panic attacks in a simple way so that anyone could understand and I came up with this analogy: I'm sure that you've all seen a pinball table, haven't you? The idea is to manoeuvre a little silver ball round various obstacles trying to avoid dropping it into the hole where it goes out of play. The first thing you have to do is put your money in the slot to set the game up. Now, think of that action as the thought or the trigger that starts off the process of your panic. Then you pull back the lever to start the ball spinning at speed round the table. The release of tension on the spring represents your adrenaline level rising, which causes the feelings of panic. You let go of the lever and all hell breaks loose. The little silver ball flies around the table, hitting barriers, ringing bells. You're in a full-blown panic attack. The ball starts to lose its momentum. Using the two buttons, which work the arm-like flippers, you try to flick the ball to keep it in play. This is you bringing in your 'what ifs' – what if this or that happens ? – adding more and more adrenaline, keeping your panic going. Keeping it in play.

But, finally, you can't control the little silver ball any longer and it drops away down the hole. You are exhausted and your body cannot maintain the level of adrenaline, so your panic automatically subsides.

I hope this helps you to understand that panic is not something that comes from 'outside', just to frighten you. When you are in a situation where you feel uneasy and scared, don't forget that it is you who will, through your anxious thoughts (triggers), pull that lever. You don't have to do it. Relax, breathe slowly and evenly, think positively, distract yourself and remember that you can stop playing emotional pinball if you really try.

Anger

We all get angry. We get angry when we feel that our illness is holding us back from doing the normal everyday things that others do. Perhaps we cannot take our children to school, go away on holiday or take a job, all because we have got this problem called anxiety, which if left to fester manifests itself into other forms of anxiety illnesses like agoraphobia, social phobia, claustrophobia, panic attacks and obsessive-compulsive disorder, to name but a few. Anger is a natural emotion but can so easily become misplaced. We get angry when we feel threatened; if things don't go the way we want them to, we feel hurt, wounded, upset. Children will stamp their feet, sulk or throw a tantrum. While we may use slightly different tactics, do we behave any differently? Perhaps we rant and rave, seethe in silence or use silence to punish the person we are angry with or bully people until they give in to our demands. If we hate a person it is likely that we hate something that we think we see in him or her that may lie within ourselves. We need to let go of anger, acknowledge that we feel angry, analyse it.

Why am I feeling angry?

Express it – find an appropriate way to let it out. Deal with it – don't forget that you are the one hurting yourself.

Strategies for dealing with anger

- Take vigorous exercise or go for a long walk.
- Throw things, provided it is safe.
- Go somewhere where you can't be heard, and yell, scream, rant and rave.
- Thump cushions and pillows.
- Count to ten before saying anything.
- Walk away from the situation if you feel yourself getting incensed.
- Show respect for the other person, he or she has feelings too.
- Work towards a win-win situation; be prepared to compromise.
- Try to defuse anger with humour.
- Work your anger through with a counsellor.
- Write your anger out, particularly if you cannot confront the person directly, especially if that person is no longer around, or has died.

Anxiety about feeling anger towards someone can often lead to a build-up of irritation and tension, which can keep a person on edge for days or weeks. That person may explode with rage completely inappropriately against others who have done nothing to incur his or her wrath. The businessman who takes a dispute with his superiors out on his wife, and the mother who is furious and vents her anger on her children because a shop assistant has been rude to her, are typical examples of this diverted rage response.

Suppression of anger in the appropriate circumstances is usually due to two main anxieties. The first is worry over how those respon-sible for the anger will react. Will they become very angry and perhaps violent themselves? Will they simply think less well of you as a result of the outburst? The second fear is that it may not be possible to control one's anger once it has been unleashed.

People who are unfamiliar with this type of emotion are often convinced that they will become 'blind with rage' and do or say something which they will greatly regret once their temper has cooled. In fact, it is much more likely that the man or woman who is constantly repressing feelings of anger will one day lose control, rather than the person who knows how to handle these emotions as a result of training and practice. Anger is only an explosive force if it is allowed to build up under pressure, but being able to lose your temper in a controlled manner can be learned. The main rule is that you should always express anger at the time and in the context to which it is appropriate. Suppressed rage always creates anxieties, either by being diverted on to innocent parties – which often leads to feelings of guilt and repentance later – or by being absorbed. Nobody makes us angry, though. We call up this destruc-tive emotion ourselves – so that means that we have the ability to change the situation, doesn't it?

4

Breathing techniques

This chapter looks at why breathing incorrectly can cause difficulties; why the way you breathe is important; and how this will help with your anxiety. It aims to help you control your breathing and practise using it to help reduce the symptoms of your anxiety.

Everyone tends to think that breathing comes naturally and that there can't be a wrong way of doing it. Unfortunately, that's not true. If, for instance, you slump on the settee in front of the TV, it may feel very comfortable but if you stay in that position for any length of time, your body will begin to ache. Sitting like that constantly could cause a lot of problems.

Breathing is the same. Breathing too rapidly for a short time won't cause too many problems, but continued rapid breathing can cause physical discomfort that can be quite frightening. As we saw in Chapter 1, this type of breathing is called hyperventilation and is a normal response to stress.

Test your breathing

As a quick test, take one hand and place it just above your navel. Place the other hand in the middle of your chest, right below the collarbone. Now, try to relax and breathe as you would normally. Which hand is moving the most? If the hand on your chest is moving most, then you are not breathing from the diaphragm. Why is this important? When you breathe primarily from the upper chest, you increase your risk of hyperventilating.

Are you a constant upper chest breather?

Perhaps you will remember doing exercises as a child and being told: 'Stand up straight, stomach in and chest out.' Being told to watch your posture and to look your best may have inadvertently created a habit of breathing mainly from the upper chest. During exercise we need to breathe more quickly to provide our muscles with oxygen to burn while we are physically active. This is how we prepare our body for action and to relieve stress by running away, for instance. However, if over-breathing becomes a habit it can cause the oxygen level in the blood to rise too much and, at the same time, the carbon dioxide level falls.

Does it really matter if I breathe from my upper chest?

Yes, it does matter and I will explain what happens. Imagine a 'U' shaped test tube. If I pour liquid into the tube it will find an equal level across both sides of the tube. Now, if I blow down one side of the tube, applying pressure to the liquid, the level will drop on that side and rise on the other. When pressure is discontinued the liquid drops to find its own level again but during this process it moves rapidly up and down, like a see-saw, until it comes to rest. This is similar to the imbalance caused by breathing incorrectly.

Does this cause a problem?

Yes, it produces all the nasty symptoms of which anxiety sufferers become afraid, such as:

- tingling in the face, hands and legs;
- muscle tremors;
- cramp;
- dizziness;
- visual problems;
- chest and stomach pains;
- exhaustion.

These symptoms are extremely alarming and cause more anxiety, then more over-breathing. The anxiety level rises even further, then the symptoms increase in what seems to be a never ending spiral.

How to reverse the situation

It is essential, therefore, that correct breathing is learned, understood and established. This is the way to get the adrenaline level lowered and under control, helping to dissipate any unpleasant feelings: breathing through the nose, both in and out, gently and evenly, filling the lungs completely. Avoid breathing from the upper chest, and use the diaphragm properly. Aim for between 8 and 12 breaths a minute (breathing in and out counts as one breath). Breathing should be smooth without gasping or gulping and it is good to concentrate on the word 'relax' as you breathe out.

How to start

Lie down flat on your back and place your hands on the area between the bottom of your ribs and your navel. Your finger tips should just be touching and as you breathe in you will feel your hands separate as your diaphragm expands. As you breathe out your finger tips will come together again. This indicates whether or not you are doing the exercise correctly. Now place your hands on your diaphragm and close your mouth and breathe in and out through your nose.

Then, as you breathe in, expand your stomach, inflate it like a balloon and as you exhale allow your stomach to deflate. Breathe to a count of 4 in and 4 out. You may not be able to manage this at first but you will be able to so with practice. What you should be aiming to do is to inflate your lungs fully and slow down your breathing to a calm, even rhythm. Control is the key thing, being able to breathe slowly and evenly to dispel all unwanted feelings.

Make yourself comfortable and then take a breath. Not too deeply: In 2 – 3 – 4 and gently out 2 – 3 – 4 and in 2 – 3 – 4 and smoothly out 2 –3 – 4 and in 2 – 3 – 4 and out 2 –3 – 4 and in (feel your stomach rise) 2 – 3 – 4 and out 2 –3 – 4, and so on.

What next?

When you have perfected the above exercise and know how your body should feel, then it is time to practise when you are sitting and, finally, when standing. Eventually, you will be able to switch to correct breathing anywhere and in any situation. By this stage you won't need to use your hands as a guide, so no one else will be aware of what you are doing. The length of time you need to do the exercise will depend on whether it is just for practice or for actually coping. For practice, once a day should suffice but when in an anxious situation, continue with the breathing exercise until the symptoms subside and the anxiety level drops.

5

Relaxation – why it's important

The importance of relaxation

Why do anxious people need to relax?

Relaxation is one of the basic building blocks needed to form a good, strong platform for recovery from any type of anxiety disorder. The pattern of nervous tension and panic which starts a circle of fear, panic and more fear needs to be broken and relaxation can go a long way to assist recovery.

When do I need to do it?

A relaxation programme needs to be done daily to keep the body calm. You need to be aware of the difference between tension and relaxation in a waking state. Although it may be pleasant, practising last thing at night and falling asleep during the programme does not teach you anything. Practise during the day when you are alert.

Why do I need to do it daily?

It has taken time for your body to become sensitized and it will take time to reverse the situation. When you first start to learn how to relax, you will probably find that it appears as if nothing is happening at all. There seems to be no improvement. Don't expect something to happen quickly – how can it when it is likely that you have been living with a high rate of tension for a long time. It takes time for the mind and body to adjust.

What has it got to do with the mind?

The mind plays an integral part: a thought can be a trigger to making you feel anxious or panicky so this has to be dealt with too when it interferes with your attempts to relax. Sometimes people are afraid to relax properly because they think they may lose control.

What do I do then?

You try again, concentrate on the word 'relax' and allow your breathing to slow down and become quiet. No doubt you will have seen a baby or small child asleep and noticed that they hardly seem to be breathing at all. The only thing that you see is a tiny movement of the diaphragm, gently up and down, quiet and even. This is what you are aiming to achieve. Get to know your body, be aware of which muscles you tend to hold tight, like hunched up shoulders, stiff legs, clenched jaw – and deliberately relax them.

Problems and getting help

When your body starts to really relax you may, during practice, get a feeling of anxiety which can make you think that you are failing. Don't give up – this is a good sign and just means that the tension is beginning to break down. This happens occasionally until the nervous system is more stable. Just relax a little more and you will quickly pass through it. You are doing well.

At this point you may need to involve a helper. If so *it is important that he or she read through the next exercises.* Your helper will need to be able to speak clearly and smoothly and in a relaxed manner, pausing regularly and allowing time to reinforce the feeling of relaxation.

Relaxation exercises

A taped version of the following is available on audiocassette from No Panic, if required (see 'Useful addresses', on page 112, for contact details). The object of these exercises is to teach you how to deeply relax your entire body by demonstrating the difference between tension and relaxation of your muscles. It is important that the exercises are done daily to achieve maximum results. Try to do the routine when you are fully aware and alert, so that you will be able to notice the difference between tension and relaxation.

Find yourself a warm, quiet room, either sitting comfortably or lying flat on your back with your eyes closed. Relax your arms by your sides and have your legs outstretched and uncrossed. It is important to focus on the word 'relax' when you are relaxing each muscle group. Try to let the relaxation happen without forcing it.

Let the feeling flow over you and deepen at its own pace. Keep your breathing shallow, calm, controlled and relaxed . . . and as you breathe out . . . relax a little more. Don't hold your breath, keep your breathing steady, regular and relaxed. Try to concentrate on the word 'relax' each time you breathe out.

What follows is a series of exercises for each major muscle group to help you learn the difference between tension and relaxation.

Hands and forearm muscles

You tense these by making fists with your hands, clenching your fists as tightly as you can and feeling the tension in your hands and forearms. So, clench your hands tight, tighter. Feel the tension in your hands and forearms . . . feel the tension . . . and relax. Relax your hands and notice the difference between tension and relaxation in your hands and forearms. Focus on the word 'relax' while letting the muscles in your hands and forearms unwind more and more deeply. Concentrate on the feeling of letting go.

Biceps (the muscles in the front of your upper arm)

You can tense these by bending your arms at the elbows and trying to touch your wrists to your shoulders. So, tense your biceps this way – tight, tighter. Feel the tension . . . hold it . . . and relax. Straighten out your arms and let them fall back to your sides and notice the difference between tension and relaxation in your biceps. Concentrate on the word 'relax' and let your biceps muscles loosen and unwind more and more deeply, and carry on that feeling of letting go. Let the muscles unwind . . . and relax. Feel them becoming more and more relaxed.

Triceps (the muscles in the back of your upper arms)

You can tense these by straightening your arms as hard as you can. So, straighten your arms hard, harder. Feel the tension . . . and relax. Relax the muscles in the back of your upper arms more and more deeply, and as you let go concentrate on the word 'relax' and just continue that feeling of relaxation throughout your arms. Let all the tension ease away. Let all the muscles of your arms loosen . . . unwind . . . and relax, noticing the difference between tension and relaxation.

Shoulder muscles

You can tense these by shrugging your shoulders, that is by drawing them up into your neck as high as you can. So, lift your shoulders high into your neck . . . high, higher. Feel the tension in your shoulders . . . feel the tension . . . and relax. Let your shoulders drop down and relax. Feel the tension ease away. And as you let your shoulders relax and unwind, concentrate on the word 'relax'. Let the muscles relax more and more deeply and carry on the feeling of letting go, noticing the difference between tension and relaxation.

Neck muscles

You can tense these by pressing your head back as hard as you can. So, press your head back and feel the tension in your neck. Feel the tension . . . hold it . . . and relax. Relax your neck and let your head rest gently back . . . no effort . . . no tension. Notice the difference between tension and relaxation in your neck. Concentrate on the word 'relax' while letting your neck relax more and more and continue the feeling of letting go. No tension in your neck.

The muscles in your forehead

You can tense these by raising your eyebrows, as though enquiring. So, raise your eyebrows and feel the tension in your forehead. Raise your eyebrows, high, higher. Feel the tension . . . hold it . . . and relax. Let your eyebrows drop and relax. Smooth out your forehead this way and notice the difference between tension and relaxation. Carry on the feeling of letting go while you concentrate on the word 'relax'.

The muscles of your brow

You can tense these by frowning as hard as you can. So, squeeze your eyebrows together and frown hard, harder. Feel the tension . . . hold it . . . and relax. Smooth out your brow and ease away the tension. Feel comfortable and relaxed and notice the difference between tension and relaxation. Focus on the word 'relax' and continue to let the muscles of your forehead unwind more and more deeply.

Eye muscles

You can tense these by squeezing your eyes tightly shut. So, squeeze your eyes tight, tighter. Feel the tension around your eyes . . . feel the tension . . . and relax. Keep your eyelids closed, resting lightly together, looking straight ahead with your eyes still. Let the tension ease away. Relax completely and continue the feeling of letting go.

Jaw muscles

You can tense these by biting your teeth together as hard as you can. So, bite your teeth together hard, harder. Feel the tension in your jaw . . . and relax. Part your teeth slightly so that there is no pressure between your teeth and feel the difference between tension and relaxation in your jaw. Feel the relief of letting go, and carry on letting your jaw loosen and relax more and more deeply while you focus on the word 'relax'.

Tongue and throat muscles

You can tense these by putting the tip of your tongue against the roof of your mouth and pushing up as hard as you can. So, push the tip of your tongue against the roof of your mouth hard, harder. Feel the tension in your tongue and throat . . . feel the tension . . . and relax. Let your tongue drop down to the bottom of your mouth . . . still and relaxed, and feel the tension ease away from your tongue and throat. Notice the difference between tension and relaxation – letting tension go, easing your tongue and throat while you concentrate on the word 'relax'.

Lip muscles

You can tense these by pressing your lips together as tightly as you can. So, press your lips together tight, tighter. Feel the tension in your lips and face . . . feel the tension . . . and relax. Relax your lips and let them rest lightly together – no pressure, gently together. Let all the tension ease away as you concentrate on the word 'relax' while you continue to let the muscles in your lips and face unwind more and more. Let your face relax completely . . . no tension in your face . . . let your muscles unwind and relax. Allow the feeling of relaxation to flow over you more and more deeply.

Chest muscles

You can tense these by taking a deep breath. So, breathe in as deeply as you can, and hold it. Feel the tension . . . feel the tension in your chest and . . . relax. Breathe right out and feel the relief of letting go. Now keep your breathing shallow, don't breathe too deeply, and notice that every time you breathe out you can relax a little more. Relax a little more each time you breathe out, and focus on the word 'relax'. No tension in your chest.

Stomach muscles

You can tense these by making your stomach hard and rigid, as though you were preparing to receive a blow. So, tense your stomach muscles tight, tighter. Feel the tension . . . feel the tension . . . and relax. Relax your stomach muscles . . . let them loosen, unwind and let go. Focus on the word 'relax' as you let the feeling of relaxation spread throughout your stomach muscles and notice the difference between tension and relaxation. Let your stomach muscles unwind more and more. Let all the tension ease away.

Hip and lower back muscles

You can tense these by arching your back and tensing your buttocks as tightly as you can. So, tense these muscles tight, tighter. Feel the tension . . . and relax. Relax your hips and your back, let all the tension ease away and notice how it feels to let the muscles loosen and relax. Focus on the word 'relax' and let the tension ease away.

Leg muscles

You can tense these by straightening your legs and pointing your toes down. So, straighten your legs to tense your thighs and point your toes down to tense your calves and feet – and feel the tension in your legs. Feel the tension . . . hold it . . . and relax. Relax your legs and let them loosen and unwind. Concentrate on the word 'relax' and notice the difference between tension and relaxation in your legs. No tension in your legs . . . let the muscles in your legs relax more and more, and notice the difference between tension and relaxation.

Relax more and more deeply, and let this feeling of relaxation spread throughout the whole of your body. Keep your breathing shallow and relaxed and every time you breathe out, relax a little more. Let the relaxation flow over you, letting all the muscles relax and unwind. No tension in your legs . . . or your hips . . . or your stomach . . . or your chest. No tension in your neck . . . or your face . . . or your shoulders . . . or your arms. Let your body feel heavy and relaxed, more and more deeply relaxed. Just feel as if you are sinking deeper and deeper.

Comfortable . . . calm . . . peaceful . . . and relaxed. No tension. Focus on the word 'relax' and enjoy the feeling of relaxation for the next few moments.

And then count backwards from four to one. When you reach one, open your eyes and sit up . . . refreshed and still feeling comfortable and relaxed.

Quick relaxation

Relax as comfortably as you can. Close your eyes and just let yourself relax and unwind. Concentrate on the word 'relax' and let the feeling of relaxation take over. Keep your breathing shallow and relaxed. Don't hold your breath, and every time you breathe out, relax a little more. Just relax as deeply as you can and let all the tensions ease away from your body. Feel comfortable and relaxed.

No tension in your hands and arms. Let your hands and arms unwind . . . completely.

No tension in your shoulders. Let your shoulders drop and relax . . . and let all the tensions ease away. No tension in your shoulders.

No tension in your neck. Let your head rest back gently and let the muscles in your neck relax . . . completely. Carry on the feeling of letting go . . . more and more relaxed.

No tension in your forehead or your brow. Smooth out your brow and let your eyebrows drop and relax.

No tension around your eyes . . . relax the muscles and let them unwind. Eyelids lightly closed, eyes looking straight ahead, more and more relaxed.

No tension in your jaw. Teeth slightly apart. No pressure between your teeth. Let your jaw relax completely. Feel the relief of letting go. More and more relaxed.

No tension in your tongue and throat. Let your tongue drop

to the bottom of your mouth and relax completely. No tension
. . . just carry on the feeling of letting go. Relax your tongue and
throat more and more.

No tension in your lips and face. Lips lightly together, no
pressure between them. Let the muscles in your face unwind
and let go. No tension in your face . . . just let it relax more and
more.

Relax the muscles in your chest. Keep your breathing shallow
and relaxed. Don't breathe too deeply, and each time you breathe
out concentrate on the word 'relax' and let your body relax a little
more.

No tension in your stomach muscles . . . let them loosen and
relax. Let all the tension in your stomach muscles ease away.
Relax completely.

Relax the muscles in your hips and back. Let them unwind
more and more. Make sure that your buttocks are completely
relaxed . . . no tension in your buttocks . . . no tension in your
hips. Just let the tension ease away.

No tension in your legs. Feel the tension ease away from your
legs and relax them completely. Let the muscles carry on relaxing
. . . more and more . . . and let the tension in your legs ease away
. . . and relax.

And continue this feeling throughout the whole of your
body. Carry on letting your body relax and unwind more and
more until you are deeply relaxed. Breathing . . . relaxed . . .
and at ease. Focus on the word 'relax' and, every time you
breathe out, relax a little more. Feel as if you are sinking deeper
and deeper, getting more and more relaxed. No tension, no
effort. Just carry on relaxing and letting go – throughout the
whole of your body. For the next few moments enjoy the
feeling of complete relaxation. Then count backwards from
four to one. When you reach one, you can either carry out the
following exercises for differential relaxation or you can open
your eyes, sit up, alert, refreshed, still feeling comfortable – and
relaxed.

Differential relaxation

While you are completely relaxed, think of the muscles in your
fingers, and move your fingers around, keeping the rest of your

body still and relaxed. Notice how it feels to move one part of your body and keep the rest completely relaxed. Then relax your hands, relax your fingers and carry on relaxing the whole of your body.

Then bend your arms at the elbows, raise your hands and make turning movements with your hands as though turning a knob. Keep the rest of your body still and completely relaxed. Turn your hands slowly from side to side. Notice how it feels to be able to move one part of your body and keep the rest completely relaxed. Carry on moving your hands from side to side and relaxing the rest of your body.

Then relax your arms again, relax your arms by your sides and let go . . . completely. Concentrate on the word 'relax' and let your whole body unwind. Let go . . . and relax.

And next, keeping the whole of your body relaxed, open your eyes, open your eyes and look around you. Look around by just moving your eyes, with the rest of your body completely relaxed. Move your eyes around and look at objects in the room and keep everything else still and relaxed . . . and notice how it feels to be able to move your eyes and keep everything else relaxed and at ease.

Then, move your head slightly from side to side and look around even further, but keep the rest of your body completely relaxed, completely at ease. No tension . . . no problems . . . just carry on moving your head and your eyes and notice how it feels to be able to move these parts of your body and keep the rest completely relaxed . . . completely comfortable. Carry on looking around you and keeping your whole body relaxed and at ease. And then, stop moving your head, and relax your head and neck completely.

Keep your eyes open but relax the muscles of your neck and keep your head still. Focus on the word 'relax' and let the relaxation flow over you.

Then, move the muscles of your tongue and jaw. Move your jaw around and move your tongue. Notice how you can move these muscles while keeping the rest of your body completely relaxed. Notice how it feels to move your jaw and tongue while keeping the rest of your body relaxed and at ease. Keep the movements smooth . . . gentle . . . and relaxed. In this way you will be able to converse using just these muscles but keeping the rest of your body calm and relaxed. Just say one or two words to see how it feels to talk while staying completely relaxed. Try saying your name . . . and once again. Say your name . . . and notice how you can talk while keeping the rest of your body relaxed and at ease. No tension, no problems. Then relax your jaw and tongue and let the whole of your body relax completely. Focus on the word 'relax' and allow yourself to unwind . . . more and more.

Next, sit up slowly with your shoulders dropped and relaxed, your neck relaxed, your stomach relaxed. Just sit relaxed and at ease. Eyes open, and sitting relaxed and comfortable. Notice how you can sit relaxed. No tension . . . comfortable and at ease.

Then, very slowly, stand up . . . stand up in a relaxed fashion, keeping the whole of your body relaxed. Face relaxed and comfortable, shoulders dropped and relaxed. Stomach and hips relaxed and at ease. Concentrate on the word 'relax' and feel how you can stand and still be at ease and relaxed. Keep your head erect and your neck relaxed.

Take a few steps around the room. Walk slowly and notice how you can walk while keeping the whole of your body relaxed. Keep the whole of the top part of your body relaxed and at ease. No tensions in your face, arms, shoulders, chest, stomach muscles or back. Breathing shallow and relaxed. Concentrate on the word 'relax' and continue to walk slowly around the room. Keep your movements loose and relaxed. Notice how you can carry out these actions and yet stay completely relaxed.

Next, pick up some small object, a book or magazine, something easy to handle, and walk around the room . . . slowly . . . while carrying this object. See how you can relax while walking and handling an object. Notice how it feels to carry out these movements while still remaining completely relaxed and at ease.

Finally, sit down again. Sit down, close your eyes and relax your entire body. Concentrate on the word 'relax' and let your body unwind . . . and let go. Remember how it felt to move while keeping the rest of your body relaxed and at ease. Continue to keep your breathing shallow and relaxed and every time you breathe out, relax a little more. Just enjoy for a few moments the feeling of letting go. Enjoy the feeling of relaxation. Feel completely relaxed, calm and at ease, and then count backwards from four to one. When you reach one, open your eyes and sit up straight – alert, refreshed, still feeling comfortable . . . and relaxed.

You have now seen how you can carry out these activities without unnecessary tension. It is possible, with practice, to increase your movements until you can carry out all sorts of tasks from housework to driving a car to playing a sport. With these relaxation techniques you will be able to deal with any situation where tension is a problem, and feel comfortable and relaxed.

6

Diet and exercise

Eating habits

The causes of anxiety and stress are complex. Some people do not eat properly due to their symptoms. Stress and anxiety can be aggravated not only by what we eat but by the way we eat. Any of the following habits can aggravate your daily level of stress:

- eating too fast or on the move;
- not chewing food at least 15–20 times before swallowing (food must be partially pre-digested in your mouth to be adequately digested later);
- eating too much, to the point of feeling bloated;
- drinking too much fluid with a meal, which can dilute stomach acid and digestive enzymes.

All the above habits put a strain on the stomach and intestines in their attempt to properly digest and assimilate foods. This adds to stress levels in two ways: directly through indigestion, bloating and cramping; indirectly through mal-absorption of essential nutrients.

Anxious people tend either to eat too little or too much. They may be so anxious that they find it difficult to swallow food. On the other hand, they may find themselves constantly 'snacking' as a form of comfort. So what can you do to change or improve your eating habits so as best to help yourself?

First and foremost, a good breakfast is essential to replenish energy. You would not expect your car to start if you had left it out, all night, with the lights on. Our 'battery' needs charging too. Keeping our blood sugar levels constant is important. If you find it difficult at first to be able to eat in the early morning, try to take just a small amount of some kind of carbohydrate – one slice of toast, a small bowl of cereal or porridge. Gradually increase the portion by, perhaps, adding sliced banana to your cereal or having two pieces of toast. So, don't go without breakfast. Charge your 'battery' ready to face the day.

If you find you are constantly snacking, then do try to have a proper meal instead, and if you feel that you need something later, make it fruit rather than chocolate or crisps. 'Grazing' can become a habit, so if you are feeling anxious, try to distract yourself by some other means. It is preferable not to eat too late in the evening, as this will not aid digestion and may not help you to get a good night's sleep.

It is known that some foods and substances tend to create additional stress and anxiety, while others promote a calmer and steadier mood. *Warning*: Before you do anything drastic about your diet, check with your GP – this is most important.

Substances that aggravate anxiety

Caffeine

Of all the dietary factors that can aggravate anxiety and trigger panic attacks, caffeine is the most notorious. You need to watch your intake of this stimulant as, for some, it can noticeably increase feelings of agitation. Many people find that they feel calmer and sleep better after they have reduced their caffeine consumption. Caffeine increases the level of the neurotransmitter norepinephrine in the brain, causing you to feel alert and awake. It also produces the very same physiological arousal response that is triggered when you are subjected to stress-increased sympathetic nervous system activity and a release of adrenaline. Too much caffeine can keep you in a chronically tense, aroused condition, leaving you more vulnerable to generalized anxiety as well as panic attacks. Caffeine contributes further to stress by causing a depletion of vitamin B^1 (thiamine), which is one of the so-called anti-stress vitamins.

Caffeine is contained not only in coffee but also in many types of tea, cola, chocolate and cocoa. If you decide to cut down on your caffeine intake, it is better to reduce it slowly so as to avoid too many withdrawal symptoms. It is possible to substitute with decaffeinated tea and coffee, which have a lower amount of caffeine.

Nicotine

Nicotine is as strong a stimulant as caffeine. It stimulates increased physiological arousal and makes the heart work harder. Smokers claim that having a cigarette 'calms the nerves', but research has proved that smokers tend to be more anxious than non-smokers, even when there are no differences in their intake of other stimulants. Smokers also tend to sleep less well than non-smokers.

Alcohol

Alcohol can become a problem, too, if it is used indiscriminately as a 'crutch'. While initially a glass or two of wine may seem to relax you and soothe your nerves, heavy, long-term drinking can actually cause anxiety, resulting in anxiety-like symptoms such as tremors, insomnia, irrational fears, palpitations and excessive sweating. Relying on alcohol to damp down anxiety symptoms can ultimately aggravate panic attacks, due to its effects on the body. Alcohol is a depressant, slowing down the central nervous system and affecting the chemistry of the brain. The jitters of a hangover do not predispose to a state of calm, not least because of the dehydration that is a prime result of over-consumption. If you enjoy a social glass or two:

- Stick to that – remember the law of diminishing returns. More alcohol won't make you feel better.
- Have plenty of water, lemonade or other mixer as well as your alcoholic drink. If you find you have drunk too much, drink plenty of water afterwards.
- Have something to eat with your drink – crisps, nuts, a sandwich, or other nibbles.

Substances that stress the body

Salt

Excessive salt stresses the body in two ways:

- it can deplete your system, and
- it raises blood pressure.

Therefore a reduction in salt intake is desirable for most people. Processed foods contain 80 per cent of the salt that is consumed in

the UK. Check the labels and look for a low salt/sodium content of
0.1g sodium per 100g, or less.

Refined sugar

Sugar has become a dirty word for many people. The fact is,
however, that the body and brain need naturally occurring sugars,
especially glucose, in order to operate. Glucose is the fuel the body
burns; it provides the energy which sustains life. Much of this
glucose is derived from carbohydrate foods: the starches in these
foods are broken down gradually into glucose. Unfortunately, these
days, we tend to eat too much *refined* sugar (and remember not just
sweets and cakes but fizzy drinks and squash come into this category), which can overload our systems too quickly and is believed
to cause a wide variety of problems, including, for some, aggravated
feelings of anxiety.

Food allergies and anxiety

An allergic reaction occurs when the body attempts to resist the
intrusion of a foreign substance. For some people, certain foods
affect the body, not only causing classic symptoms such as a runny
nose, mucus and sneezing but a host of psychological or psychoso-
matic symptoms, including any of the following:

- anxiety or panic,
- depression or mood swings,
- dizziness,
- irritability,
- insomnia,
- headaches,
- confusion and disorientation,
- fatigue.

Such reactions occur in many individuals only when they eat an
excessive amount of a particular food, a combination of offending
foods, or have excessively low resistance due to a cold or infection.
Other people are so highly sensitive that only a small amount of
the wrong food can cause debilitating symptoms. Often the subtler,
psychological symptoms have a delayed onset, making it difficult to
connect them with the offending foods.

Food allergies can definitely be a contributing factor to excessive anxiety and mood swings for certain people. If you suspect this to be a problem, consult a State Registered Dietician.

It is not always easy to identify which, if any, of the many elements in food and/or drugs might be inducing or aggravating anxiety or stress, but it is certainly advisable to check your dietary and drug intake. When all is taken into consideration, following a healthy, balanced diet is a very sensible option.

Exercise

Exercise can help with anxiety, but the sad truth is that many people with anxiety, panic and related disorders find that their condition stops them being able to take exercise. If you are able to get out and about, it obviously makes it easier for you to exercise. A daily walk at a steady pace that will get your circulation going, will also lower your adrenaline level. But for some, this isn't possible. Agoraphobia may prevent them leaving home, for example, or the fear of a panic attack may mitigate against, say, going for a nice long walk, or taking a swim. It may be that joining a club of some sort, tennis or squash for instance, or going to the gym, is not possible at present, due to your anxiety problem. However, you could include this in your recovery programme as a target to aim for in the future.

Meanwhile, if you are unfortunate enough not to be able to take regular exercise because you cannot leave your home, this section looks at simple, gentle exercises to do at home.

Exercising at home

There is still a lot you can do to help yourself. The following exercises are simply to keep you flexible and give you a feeling of well-being. It is important, though, that you check with your doctor that they are suitable for you. Take things easily and sensibly. If at any point you feel pain or dizziness, stop. Don't try too hard and don't overdo it.

Using a chair

A strong dining chair that supports the back is recommended, and your feet should touch the floor in a natural position. When you are seated, the whole of your upper leg should be supported by the seat, your feet should be slightly apart and flat on the floor.

Bend your arms so that your hands come upwards to touch your shoulders.

Stretch your arms forward at shoulder level and then back again to touch your shoulders.

Move your arms from the shoulder position out to the side and back again to the shoulders.

Next, from the shoulder position, take your arms up straight above your head – but only as far as it feels comfortable. Try not to lift your shoulders, keep them down. Return to the shoulder position.

Take your arms down to your sides.

Supporting one leg with both hands under the thigh, lift the leg and stretch it forwards. Allow the leg to lift to the horizontal position or until tension is felt. Do not force it.

Repeat with the other leg.

Standing position

The first five movements in the sitting position (described above) can be done standing if preferred. If you feel a little unsteady when standing it is helpful to have a solid support beside you, a table for instance, so that you can put out a hand to correct your balance if necessary.

From the upright position, feet comfortably apart, keeping your back straight, slowly bend your knees and then slowly return to the upright position.

Using the table or the back of a chair to help you balance, swing one leg forwards and backwards. Keeping your back and your other leg straight, swing from the hip.

Repeat the exercise with your other leg.

These exercises can be done daily, increasing the amount of times each movement is done, as you progress. Do remember to take it easy to start with, especially if you are trying them on your own.

Using the stairs

If getting out of breath makes you feel anxious, then try walking up the stairs, slowly at first and then increasing the rate you ascend until you are able to run up without worrying. This could become part of your recovery programme, especially if you are afraid of hyperventilating.

7

Anxiety and phobias

We've talked at some length about the mechanisms of panic, and about anxiety in general. However, what about related problems? When does general anxiety turn into specific phobias, and how do you know if you've got a phobia? (though to most people it's all too obvious). Most importantly, what can you do about them? This chapter looks at what exactly a phobia is; what anxiety is and why we feel it; the connection between anxiety and fear; how a 'phobic' person differs from a 'normal' one; and the facts about the main kinds of severe anxiety disorders. The aim is to help you check whether your ideas about phobias are correct and decide whether it *is* a phobia that is affecting you.

What is a phobia?

I am going to explain about phobias and help you decide whether the problems that you have experienced are actually a phobia. But first, here is a story about a person with a phobia.

Karen: It was a pleasant sunny day in Parktown. Spring was in the air. The leaves were green. Birds were singing and bees were buzzing in the lilac trees. People were strolling along past No. 28 on their way to the shops. Next door, old Mrs Goodheart was sitting out in the garden with her cat. Karen looked out of her window and saw a bus full of people trundle past. She needed to do some shopping herself but thinking about it made her feel unsettled. Her throat somehow started to feel dry. She reluctantly made a list – something from the butcher, a newspaper, a few things from the grocer, some fruit and vegetables.

As she opened the door she felt a sudden flip as her heart missed a beat. She looked down and saw her hands were trembling. 'What's wrong with me?' she wondered.

As Karen left the house and got out into the street she started to feel quite bad. She went hot and cold all over and, in spite of the lovely spring sunshine, the trembling got worse and her pulse was racing madly. It was almost like a horror film – she felt as though some invisible monster was creeping up on her and getting nearer and nearer . . . At the end of the street the feeling was so overpowering that Karen was convinced she was going to faint, or scream out in panic.

The only thing she could think of was getting back to the safety of home as quickly as she could. She turned and, clutching her shopping bag in a vice-like grip, she walked back as fast as possible without drawing attention to herself. She didn't stop until she had slammed the front door behind her. Then she sat down and burst into tears. 'What's happening to me? I don't understand!' she cried.

Karen's problem was agoraphobia but it could have been one of the many different 'specific' phobias – of birds, cats, wind, thunder, and so on – or a mixture of these. No doubt you have experienced something similar yourself. Phobias are much more common than most people imagine. Even so, few people really understand what phobias are, and a lot of people have completely the wrong idea. Here are some ideas about what phobias are and what sort of people they affect. Note any of them that you agree with.

Phobias are:

(a) just imagination – the sort of thing that silly women with nothing better to do often complain about;
(b) a kind of mental illness;
(c) a disease;
(d) all in the mind;
(e) a sign that someone is starting to go mad;
(f) a kind of handicap;
(g) something you can easily catch from other people;
(h) something that only weak people get;
(i) a set of bad habits that are hard to shake off;
(j) a severe kind of anxiety;
(k) something that doctors aren't interested in;
(l) rather rare.

Now, here are my comments about that mixed bag of ideas about phobias:

(a) Phobias are just imagination: NO. The fears that cause them may be imaginary but the feelings that phobias create are only too real.

(b) Phobias are a kind of mental illness: NO. They are something that affects the mind but they are quite different from mental illnesses like schizophrenia, epilepsy or depression (though having a phobia for a long time can make people feel depressed).

(c) Phobias are a disease: NO. They are not 'organic' like arthritis or high blood pressure and they are not caught by a 'bug', like measles, TB or AIDS.

(d) Phobias are all in the mind: NO. They affect the mind because they affect the way we feel, but they are basically about the way we behave and they involve the body as well as the brain.

(e) Phobias are a sign of madness: NO. As I've already said, a phobia is not a mental illness and there is no evidence that people with phobias get mental illnesses, any more than other people do.

(f) Phobias are a kind of handicap: YES. In many ways they have more in common with restricted vision, or being confined to a wheelchair. A phobia is a condition that prevents people from doing the ordinary everyday things that most people do.

(g) Phobias are something you can catch: NO. You catch a cold but not a phobia – though some people copy their parents' phobias in the same way they copy their smoking or drinking habits.

(h) Phobias are something only weak people get: NO. Anyone can have a phobia and many 'strong personalities' with lots of self-confidence are also affected.

(i) Phobias are bad habits: YES. This is much more like it – phobias are a self-damaging way of behaving that has become a habit. Unfortunately, the phobic habit tends to be deeply ingrained and therefore hard to get rid of merely by 'an effort of will'.

(j) Phobias are a severe kind of anxiety: YES. The phobic reaction is basically a fear reaction and fear is only anxiety in a stronger form.

(k) Phobias are something doctors are not interested in: NO. Most family doctors are interested and would like to help but, like the rest of us, they find phobic conditions frustrating because there is no simple cure.

(l) Phobias are rare: NO. They are very common.

To sum up:

- Phobias are common.
- They handicap people – often severely.
- They are not a disease but a condition in which people experience strong feelings of fear in situations that are not really dangerous at all.
- Reacting this way soon becomes a deeply ingrained habit – a conditioned way of behaving which is very hard to shake off.

It can't just be anxiety, can it?

People with phobias often feel so bad in so many different ways that they can't believe that this dreadful affliction is simply caused by anxiety. But it is – phobias are a form of anxiety, though it may be anxiety of a very severe kind. Ordinary mild anxiety is something everyone has now and again: Will I get there on time? Will John be angry with me for spending all that money? He's taking this bend too fast! I've got to complain about this new carpet! The boss wants to see me – am I in trouble? I've got to make a report to the committee tonight.

Outright fear is a fairly common experience too – when a car goes out of control, or someone threatens you with violence or an aggressive dog comes charging up to you. If you think about it, you can see that mild anxiety and sheer terror are only different points on the same scale:

LOW → HIGH

Mild anxiety	*Moderate anxiety*	*Severe anxiety/fear*	*Sheer terror*
I think there may be a fierce dog around here somewhere.	That dog is giving me a funny look.	That dog is baring its teeth and snarling at me.	The dog is actually attacking me.

As you can see, 'anxiety' shades into 'fear' but it's not possible to say exactly where. That's because there isn't any real difference between anxiety and fear – they are basically just different degrees of the same thing. There is one important difference though: for most people, anxiety is about what might happen and fear is what you feel when it does.

If you have a phobia, you may be surprised to learn that fear is often a good thing. Indeed, it is hard to see how human beings could have survived as a species if we had no fear. After all, we are soft-bodied, fairly weak and slow moving – no match for a hungry tiger in a fight, for example.

Different types of anxiety phobias

Agoraphobia

Generally, agoraphobic people find it very difficult or even impossible to carry out certain activities that threaten their sense of safety. If you think you may be agoraphobic, do any of these feelings reflect your experience?

- feeling very anxious when you are in a place where you feel 'trapped' and from which you cannot easily 'escape',
  - in crowded or public places,
  - in a lift,
  - on public transport,
  - standing in a queue,
  - on a bridge,
  - sitting in the dentist's or hairdresser's;
- feeling you need to have a companion to help you go out, and then becoming totally reliant on this person;
- feeling worse the further you get from the 'safety' of home;
- feeling that if you can't escape from a situation where you feel anxious you will panic and lose control.

Agoraphobia is a serious handicap for a large number of people – though no one knows exactly how many are actually confined to their homes by their condition. People used to think of it as being 'fear of open spaces', but this is not right. Agoraphobia is usually a fear of being trapped or marooned somewhere far from the 'safety' of home. This may be a busy shopping centre, or a bridge, or an unfamiliar part of town. Indeed, we often refer to 'the agoraphobic cluster' because people with this condition often find they have a collection of different but related problems.

Those people who have a particular difficulty with large open areas may be affected by the specific problem of Space Phobia. Agoraphobic people often also have similar fears to social phobics –

for example: blushing, trembling or doing something embarrassing when talking, eating or writing in public.

Agoraphobia usually affects people first between the ages of 16 and 35 and can come on suddenly or gradually. Often it is preceded by a series of 'life stresses' which cause anxiety to build up and reduce self-confidence; however, it doesn't often seem to be related to a single shock or 'trauma'.

It can come and go for months or years before becoming a permanent problem but, once it has been present continuously for a year or more, it may persist for a long time unless treated. The symptoms of agoraphobia vary greatly and often those affected manage to tolerate it for many years. However, it does have a tendency to worsen rapidly once it has become established. Where the anxiety is relatively low the symptoms can include palpitations, feelings of nausea and chest pains. As it becomes more severe there may be difficulty in breathing, dizziness, a feeling of being 'unreal', 'jelly legs', intense sweating, faintness and restricted sight and hearing. At its most serious the person affected may experience a strong feeling that he or she is about to go mad or die (the panic reaction). In the longer term, agoraphobics' other symptoms may include: depression; obsessive thoughts; loss of interest in sex.

If you identify with several of the feelings listed above, you may have agoraphobia. Do talk with your doctor.

General anxiety disorder (GAD)

Phobias are fears of particular objects, creatures or situations but people with GAD feel anxious in virtually every situation. They may worry endlessly about the health and safety of their family, about the future, about their job. This may lead them to feel that they are going mad, but this is not so. Once again, it is anxiety and it boils down to the way the person's whole system has been conditioned to behave. Depression can be an important cause of general anxiety, even if it is concealed. To a person whose overall 'energy level' is lowered by depression, the world is a very anxious place where problems grow out of all proportion.

Obsessive-compulsive disorder (OCD)

Like phobias, this condition is a form of anxiety, but on the surface it may seem very different. Forms of OCD vary greatly (see Chapter 10), but frequent repetitive rituals such as endless washing, counting and checking (taps, light switches, doors, etc.) are typical. People with OCD realize the rituals are senseless and futile but feel helpless to resist the compulsion to perform them. They may avoid any situation thought to be 'dirty', or may wash themselves and their clothes over and over again.

Others have to perform special rituals before completing some ordinary action like going to bed or coming indoors. The rituals can take hours, because if somehow they aren't quite 'right' they have to be done all over again from the beginning. Hoarding, searching for invisible but possibly dangerous objects, and obsessive thoughts all occur – all provoked by some deep underlying anxiety.

Specific phobias

These are persistent irrational fears of particular objects, creatures or situations, arising when close to such objects and producing a very strong desire to avoid them. The person affected almost always recognizes that their reaction is out of all proportion to the 'threat' posed by the thing they fear – but this makes no difference.

Many people have a strong dislike of things like spiders and snakes, of being shut in, of dentists or of being too close to cliff edges, and avoid them when it is reasonable to do so. Phobics, however, are drastically over-sensitized to these 'triggers'. Thus someone with a phobia about scissors may often have a strong anxiety reaction to a picture of a pair of scissors or even just the thought of scissors.

Fortunately, although specific phobias are common, they are not usually as crippling as agoraphobia and social phobia. Londoners who are phobic about travelling in the Underground, for example, can go by bus instead; and although a fear of wasps, for instance, is very unpleasant at least it is only seasonal. The commonest types of specific phobia reported to No Panic include: bees, birds, blood, cats, crane flies, darkness, dentists, dogs, driving, heights, hospitals, illness and death, injections, pigeons, snakes, space, spiders, wasps, wind and weather.

Social phobias

These are a broad group of phobias that all seem to have in common a fear of being the centre of attention and of then behaving in an embarrassing or humiliating way. It can be seen as a kind of extreme self-consciousness. Typical situations feared (and therefore avoided) include: speaking, eating or drinking in public; using a public lavatory; preparing food, drink, or even writing, while being watched. The fears tend to be strongest in unfamiliar places, but they can occur at home when visitors, especially strangers, are present.

What those affected usually fear is that other people will notice how anxious they are feeling – the trembling voice or hands, the furious blushing, etc. This creates a vicious circle which increases their anxiety and makes it even more noticeable: then there is a 'genuine' reason for feeling even more anxious in future.

Like other phobics, social phobics have a strong compulsion to avoid the situation that makes them anxious and embarrassed. This gives another twist to the spiral of avoidance and sensitivity.

What exactly is your problem?

What really makes people frightened isn't always what it first seems. The aim of this section is to help you work out exactly what makes you anxious and to encourage you to talk to your GP about what you are going through.

A broad look at the problem

Have you a fairly clear idea of what category of anxiety condition is affecting you? Perhaps you are agoraphobic – this is the biggest single group. Alternatively you may have General Anxiety Disorder, a social problem, or one of the many specific phobias. You may even be obsessive or compulsive, although this is less common.

It might be that you are affected by a combination of several of these anxiety problems. Agoraphobics often have social phobias and specific phobias too. What is more confusing is that severe social phobia, or maybe a specific phobia perhaps of thunder, lightning, strong winds, birds or insects may have roughly the same result – the person affected feels strongly inclined to stay at home where he or she feels 'safe'.

I would like you to write down on a sheet of paper *broadly* what you consider your anxiety problem to be. After you have done that, note down the five situations that make you feel most anxious.

Getting below the surface

I asked you for a broad description of your anxiety problem and we'll assume that what you wrote down is correct. However, it is quite easy to be mistaken about what is *really* triggering your anxieties. Here are two examples of what I mean.

Example 1: Marie

For a long time, Marie had been frightened of certain kinds of insects. Not bees, wasps or house flies, but grasshoppers, crane flies and suchlike. If she saw locusts or praying mantises on TV wildlife programmes she would scream and run out of the room. It seemed clear enough: she was phobic about insects of the long and narrow type. She drew up a self-exposure programme to deal with this problem and at first it went quite well. She kept a dead crane fly in a small bottle and, after a while, felt quite relaxed about having it in her handbag. But then on holiday touring Scotland that September she had two panic attacks. The first was at a small fishing port, the other was out in the country where the farmer was using a 'combine' to harvest the corn. At first this was a great mystery but Marie soon realized that it couldn't just be the insects which made her anxious – there was more to it than that.

Here are small sketches of the things that made Marie feel panicky. What would you say they had in common?

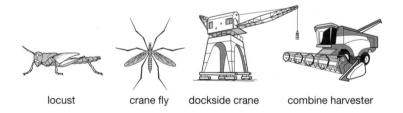

locust   crane fly   dockside crane   combine harvester

Did you realize what the underlying problem was? Not dockside cranes, combine harvesters or insects as such, but things that were a certain shape. Who knows what originally sensitized Marie to this particular shape. Perhaps it was seeing a film of the sinister claw of a praying mantis waiting to strike. (It is quite a frightening idea – as the insect-like monsters in the film *Aliens* demonstrate.) Perhaps it was a silly children's game – but the cause doesn't really matter.

The important thing was to find out precisely what would trigger her fears because her insect-based exposure programme wasn't doing the trick. She needed a programme based around a variety of objects with that particular shape.

Example 2: Kieran

Kieran, a young single man with severe anxiety problems, explained to his psychologist that he was afraid of noises at night. He lived alone in a flat in an old house and if he heard a creak or rattle from downstairs it used to make him sick with anxiety, so that he couldn't get to sleep for hours wondering and thinking about the possible cause. But after talking about it at some length and trying to work out a self-exposure programme based around noises, he began to feel that maybe noises were not the main problem.

We don't know enough about Kieran to be sure what was really troubling him, but can you think of a more likely explanation than 'noises'? As I said, we'd need to go into Kieran's case much more deeply to be confident of fully understanding it, but it seems likely that being alone, especially at night, was the main problem. Obviously, if he tried to desensitize himself to noises, that wouldn't do the trick. It would not solve his fear of being alone and afraid during the night.

What about you?

These two examples show that it's important to work out exactly what your anxiety problem consists of and this may mean digging below the surface, because the answer isn't always obvious. So now think carefully about yourself.

Do you fear 'going out'? Or is it really a fear of:

- being alone?
- being far from home?
- having a sudden illness?
- collapsing and dying?
- meeting strangers?
- something else out there (say, wind, birds or dogs)?

Do you fear 'people'? Or is it really a fear of:

- humiliating yourself (trembling or fainting)?
- being attacked?
- attacking someone else?
- being so ugly or ridiculous that someone will notice?

You are now going to make a really accurate statement of what exactly makes you anxious. The way to work this out is first to double-check the five objects or situations that make you feel most anxious and which you listed previously. Is that list still right, do you think? If so, write those five things down. (If not change the list now.) You might well list situations like: being in a crowded shop; eating in a restaurant; having to travel on a bus; having to go near a dog, and so on.

The second stage is to work out what it is about these situations that causes you a problem. For example:

- In a crowded shop you might fear being trapped inside if there was a fire.
- In a restaurant you might fear being ignored or humiliated by the waiter; you might even fear choking or vomiting up your food and making a spectacle of yourself.
- On a bus you might fear being unable to get to the door in time for your stop, or perhaps fear that the bus will crash or topple over.
- With a dog you might fear that the dog will chase you and cause you to run into the traffic and get hurt.

Look back to where I asked you to write down what you considered your problem to be, in broad terms. Now think about it again in the light of what I have just been saying. What *really* frightens you in the five situations you listed? Note down your considered version of 'Situations that make me anxious' and 'Things that *really* make me anxious in those situations'. Obviously, it is important to be as accurate and truthful as possible. The most important part of recovery – the self-exposure (see Chapter 8), which is yet to come – may not work properly if you don't get these issues straight at this stage.

Getting medical advice

Most people with phobias do not get treatment of any kind, and of those who do go to their family doctor, many do not get the 'cure' they were expecting. In fact, you can't expect your GP to cure you, but you can expect to receive help, and of course most GPs really want to help, even if they are busy and even if they can't see an easy solution. Have you spoken to your doctor?

If you haven't spoken to your GP in the last few months, we strongly recommend you do so soon. Make an appointment, explain your problem, explain that you are planning to follow this self-therapy and ask what help can be provided.

Why you should see your GP

- GPs are concerned with all aspects of your health and they will want to be sure that your anxiety isn't complicated by some other medical condition.
- If you are being prescribed drugs, especially tranquillizers, the doctor may suggest reducing the dose to help you make progress with your self-exposure treatment.
- On the other hand, if you aren't taking tranquillizers and you're very anxious, your GP may prescribe small doses to help you make the more difficult steps in your self-exposure programme.
- If your case is very severe, your doctor should know about it: he or she may refer you to a clinical psychologist for therapy (you should accept this if you get the chance).
- If you are dependent on drugs (including tranquillizers) or alcohol you may need help in reducing the dependency before you can get your self-exposure programme started.
- If you are depressed, self-exposure is difficult; however, depression isn't easy to self-diagnose: feeling depressed isn't necessarily the same as being clinically depressed. If you wake up each morning with panics that take hours to disappear, if you only feel better in the evenings and if you are off your food and losing weight, depression may be the cause. You may need medication.

The golden rule is: keep your GP informed. It won't do any harm and it may do some good. He or she will be pleased that you are doing something for yourself. And remember: *You* may think you are phobic, Betty at the corner shop may think you are phobic: but only a qualified medical person can give you a definite diagnosis. The same applies to any form of anxiety, including OCD. A medical diagnosis will reassure you that your problem really is anxiety based.

8

Self-help for phobias

Introducing self-treatment – self-exposure work

Earlier I explained that most people learn to cope with anxiety by facing up to the things that make them anxious, thus making themselves less sensitive to fear – but that phobics somehow take a wrong turning and learn that anxiety goes away if they avoid the things that make them anxious. They then become conditioned to produce the fear response at the slightest provocation. Well, self-treatment gets you to do exactly what 'normal' people do – face up to your anxieties. This means deliberately going into the situation where you feel anxious, until you become less sensitive; then going a bit further and becoming less sensitive still, until you can cope with situations that were once quite impossible for you.

What you are doing is putting the conditioning process in reverse: 'retraining your stupid bodyguard' to behave more sensibly and let you back into normal life again. As I have said, fear is like a bully and the best way to deal with it is to face up to it. Self-exposure treatment means doing just that – exposing yourself to your fears – and it will definitely cause you some uncomfortable moments. You will have to deliberately do things that make you feel anxious. But, the good news is that no one expects you to go straight into the ring with the big bully.

Instead, you are going to undertake a training programme so that you can get there in easy stages. Just like someone training to be an athlete or a boxer, you will need to work at it but you can gradually make yourself tougher and stronger and more confident, until you are fit enough to take on your worst fears. On the way there, you will dispose of some of your lesser fears quite easily.

Self-check

Find one word to complete these sentences correctly.

1 Anxiety is something that ? experiences from time to time.

2 Both anxiety and fear are often ? because they protect us from danger.

3 Both anxiety and fear cause the drug ? to be released into our bloodstream.

4 A phobia is anxiety plus ?

5 The commonest single kind of phobia is ?

6 There is no miracle ? for phobia.

7 There is little to be gained from seeking out the ? of your phobia.

The answers are on page 61, but try and complete the above before looking! How well did you do? Go back through the list again if you got several of them wrong.

Planning exposure and setting goals for phobias

You have built a wall of negativity with fears and 'what ifs' and now it is time to start using a ladder of recovery to climb over that wall. What you must do is to prepare yourself physically and mentally for the forthcoming effort:

- You must learn how to control your breathing to minimize the symptoms of panic.
- You have to learn how your body should feel when it is in a relaxed state.
- You must look at your diet and eating habits to see how they are affecting your well-being.
- You must think about your self-esteem, is it so low that it is almost non-existent?

It may be an idea to keep a diary to record progress.

Decision time: when, where and how are you going to start climbing your ladder, actually trying out your plans, practising and using the skills you have learned? It will be a great moment when you put your head above the parapet. How are you going to do that? First you have to decide the length of the ladder you might need. What is your ultimate goal? It must be specific. How are you going to get your feet on the first rung? Don't make it impossible to reach. Consider carefully and work out a practical and attainable first challenge. You may want to discuss this with someone who understands and has empathy with your problem. Write down your goal in your diary and keep a record of what you did and how you felt when you attempted to get on the first rung of your ladder.

Where are you headed?

You should by now be reasonably clear about what situations and objects trigger your fears. An old Chinese proverb says: 'The longest journey starts with a single step.' This is good common sense. If you travel a long distance you don't start your journey in the middle, you start at the beginning and travel through all the places en route. You set out from your base covering the first mile before you start to cover the second and so on. There is also an English proverb which states: 'Don't try to run before you can walk,' and that is relevant too.

So what is all this about? Well, it's about the journey you have to make in order to overcome your fears and do the things that you want to do but can't. You are going to take it a step at a time and the steps have got to be manageable ones. However, this is a journey and you are not just wandering about at random, so the first thing to do is to decide where you want to go.

Choosing specific goals

Your goals will be your objectives – the targets you want to achieve. Everyone who has an anxiety disorder will quite possibly have different aims, for example:

'I want to be able to travel on public transport whenever I need to.'
'I want to be able to walk with the kids to school without panicking.'
'I want to be able to go shopping at the supermarket on my own.'

'I want to be able to stroke a cat.'
'I want to be able to go to the dentist.'
'I want to be able to go to pubs and parties like my friends.'

Notice that these goals are quite specific, that is they talk about particular things that a person wants to do. It is no good making vague statements like, 'I would like to live a normal life' or 'I want to feel better than I do at the moment.' The reason for being specific is that it is much easier to plan your journey, and much easier to tell whether you are getting there or not. In other words, specific goals let you measure your progress.

The goals you set should be related to the frightening situations that you listed, the precise things that frighten you. Thus in one of the examples I gave earlier, Marie who was frightened by crane-shaped things of all sizes, might set one of her goals as: 'I want to be able to walk past the big building site down the road without running away.'

How many goals will you set yourself? Perhaps it will be five – but the number could easily be either smaller or greater. Some people with specific phobias will only have one goal, like Marie. Agoraphobics and people with social phobias will usually have several. Don't feel obliged to set five goals just because I have suggested that number, but do try to make sure that your goals are genuinely different ones, not versions of the same thing.

Think carefully and then write down what your own personal goals will be. Make sure they are specific and that they cover the exact things that frighten you. Are you sure you've got that right? It's very important, because otherwise your self-exposure work may take you in the wrong direction.

The steps on the way

Right. You've set your goals, so you know where your journey is taking you. Next you need to list all the principal places you're going to pass through on the way. These are the stages in your self-exposure programme, the steps on your journey to recovery.

Here is a typical example of the steps for Mrs D., a severe agora-phobic: Mrs D. would really like to be able to go shopping in the town centre but this is unrealistic, she can't even get to the shop at the corner of her street at the moment. So her initial goal is 'to be able to walk to the shop at the corner of the street without help'. Working with a helper, she decided on five steps, each of which represented a more difficult task than the previous one. The steps broke the journey down into manageable stages – she couldn't make the leap straight to Step 3, because that was just too difficult for her, so Steps 1 and 2 were included to help her get there.

Step 1   Walk to the shop at the corner of the street with a helper.
Step 2   Walk to the shop with the helper following 50 yards behind.
Step 3   Walk to the shop with the helper following 100 yards behind.
Step 4   Walk to the shop with the helper waiting at the shop.
Step 5   Walk to the shop without the helper.

Your steps need to be in the right order and this depends not on distance but on how difficult the steps are. An agoraphobic person may feel:

- fairly anxious about going to the public library a mile away;
- less anxious about going to the shops half a mile away;
- very anxious about a footbridge at the end of the street.

If this is so, then in the list of steps the shops should come before the library and the library before the footbridge (though don't forget it is always possible that the difficulty with the footbridge could be a different kind of phobia).

How much anxiety?

Self-exposure steps are all about facing up to anxiety and becoming less sensitized to the things that make you anxious: you do have to experience anxiety for this work. But though your programme of steps represents a rising scale of difficulty, that doesn't mean you will feel more and more anxious as you go on. On the contrary: right now you may feel that Step 5 is going to be a lot more difficult than Step 1, but once you've dealt with Step 1 you will have already reduced your *total* level of anxiety and Step 2 won't seem so bad. The same will apply as you move from Step 2 to Step 3.

Also, you are not being asked to face more anxiety than you can stand. All the research on this subject shows that though you do have to experience some anxiety in order to overcome it, you don't have to experience a vast amount. A moderate amount of anxiety will do the trick, and that is the whole point of doing exposure in easy stages.

Here is another example, showing some of the steps that a person with driving phobia might take – the goal is to be able to make long-distance trips alone.

Step 1   Sit in the car with the engine running.
Step 2   Drive a few yards up the road, switch off the engine then walk back (if necessary, kick the car and curse it) – the watching neighbour will think it has broken down and someone else can bring it back later.
Step 3   Work up to driving round the block.
Step 4   Try a longer journey with a 'co-driver' sitting beside you.
Step 5   Try a longer journey on your own.
Step 6   Try a journey on a 'trapping' road like a motorway, again with a co-driver beside you.
Step 7   As Step 6 – but alone.

Here is another example of a programme of self-exposure steps, this time for someone with a specific phobia about cats. However, I have muddled up the steps. Can you put them in the right order? Decide what order they should come in and check your answers with those on page 61.

(a) Look at black and white photographs of cats.
(b) Look at videos of cats.
(c) Draw a rough cat shape on a small piece of paper.
(d) Step further towards the cats inside the open doorway.
(e) Look at larger coloured photographs of cats.
(f) Look at real cats through a closed window.
(g) Increase the size of your drawings and make them more lifelike.
(h) Look through a partly opened window then open it wider and wider.
(i) Look at cats through an open doorway.

Of course, this particular programme of steps wouldn't work for everyone. Cats are friendly and inquisitive and may come running towards you, so an alternative would be to have a helper who would restrain the cat (on their lap or in a basket), then the self-exposure steps would be about getting closer and closer until you could touch it. You might also have to think carefully about what sort of cats frighten you. All cats? Big cats? Ginger cats? If it was all cats, you might need to make sure that the ones you were exposed to represented a wide selection, otherwise you might find yourself being quite happy with a polite Siamese but still highly sensitized to ginger moggies.

A summary of the rules

Before you decide on the steps for your personal 'journey', here is a summary of the rules:

Rule one: The steps should be like steps on a ladder – don't make them so steep or so far apart that they are too difficult for you to manage. In particular, don't make the first step too big.

Rule two: Each step must be higher than the last so that you are really making headway. A step that doesn't raise your level of anxiety isn't getting you anywhere.

Rule three: Fit in as many steps as you need to reach your goal (some ladders are longer than others and if you are very frightened, the steps may need to be closer together).

Rule four: Steps can be measured in time as well as distance – a step can be something like staying in a situation that makes you anxious for ten minutes when you could only manage five minutes before.

Rule five: Every step is a valuable achievement in itself.

Your steps to your goals

You should now be ready to draw up your list of steps to reach your goals. Think carefully about the examples I have given and the five rules. Start with the first goal on your list. Write it down as 'Goal No. 1' and write down a list of steps you will take to achieve that goal (use as many steps as you believe you will need): 'Step 1', 'Step 2', and so on. You will need to draw up a list like this for all the separate goals you intend to tackle and all the steps you need to take to reach each of those goals. Then all you have to do is work your way through them.

But what about getting some help? If you're ready to begin, go straight to Chapter 13, 'Getting help and support from others', to see how family and friends can support you as you work your way to your goals. If your problem is obsessive-compulsive disorder, you might find it helpful first to read the next four chapters, which deal specifically with OCD.

Answers to 'self-check' questions on page 55:
1 everyone; 2 useful; 3 adrenaline; 4 avoidance; 5 agoraphobia; 6 cure; 7 cause.

Answers to 'Steps' quiz on page 59:
The correct order is: 1 (c); 2 (g); 3 (a); 4 (e); 5 (b); 6 (f); 7 (h); 8 (i); 9 (d).

9

Obsessive-compulsive disorder (OCD)

I want to start off immediately by challenging the mystery that sometimes seems to cloud obsessive-compulsive disorder. OCD is an anxiety disorder that is no different from any other anxiety state or phobia, in the sense that without the basis of fear there would be no illness.

Understanding OCD

The fear factor

As we saw in Chapter 2, we need a certain amount of fear to survive – but anxiety disorders, including OCD, are really examples of fear that has got out of hand.

Anxiety disorders – mainly OCD, panic and phobias – are all related to the human body's nervous system and its reaction to fear. We all get frightened at times, and we all react in a very similar manner to a frightening experience, whether we have anxiety disorders or not (for example, if you've ever been in or narrowly avoided a traffic accident). When we have a 'scare', our heart beats quicker, we sweat, tremble and some people faint or have hysterics. Fear protects us – without it we would just walk into the middle of the road. So, you can see that we are not born with an inbuilt knowledge of 'fear', we have to learn it as we grow up. 'Fear' is a vital part of common sense and is used daily to survive, even though we may not realize it. Just stop and ponder that point the next time you step off a pavement without thinking!

The problem for people with OCD, as for others with an anxiety disorder, is that they have learned too much 'fear'. Consequently they get messages of 'fear' when there is nothing to be frightened of. They might be 'afraid' that they haven't washed their clothes, hands or work surfaces enough, that they haven't checked the gas taps or light switches properly, or that the front door is not locked securely. I'm sure everyone can think of times when this has happened to them in some minor way. Is it any wonder that OCD is known as the 'doubting' illness? People with OCD are never 100 per cent sure that things have been done correctly. So, what to most people is a simple task, such as checking that a door is locked, is a mammoth job to those with OCD. They can't quite convince themselves that the door is fastened securely, and consequently go back time and time again to check. Sometimes this can take several hours. The small feeling of alarm that we might experience, if it occurs to us that we may have left a door unlocked, is nothing by comparison with the continual, nagging worry that blights the life of a person with OCD. The feelings of those with OCD are very real and distressing and have to be dealt with, usually by doing, saying or thinking something which reduces the amount of doubt or fear they experience.

Thus, 'fear' takes over the person's life and is a continual problem – but people with anxiety disorders are not mad, insane or schizophrenic, neither will they become so, as was explained in Chapter 3. The problem is one of neurosis, not psychosis.

Crossed wires

Sometimes it is easier to explain the problems and difficulties of OCD by using simple analogies. Do you remember the old type of telephone switchboard where an operator had to plug in the incoming call? If you are not old enough to remember then I'm sure you've seen one in films. It consisted of a board which had many connections, and as an outside call came through, the operator would answer and then plug the caller into the appropriate connection. The connecting wires crossed and interlaced like spaghetti on a plate. Sometimes, the operator would get flustered and plug the wrong wire into the wrong connection, and consequently the wrong people were linked together, not knowing each other and completely baffled by the conversation.

This is what happens to a person suffering from OCD. A trigger thought (phone ringing) comes into the mind and due to a bleep in transmission (wrong connection) the person (the operator) hears an odd and strange message, which is of course the crossed line. These thoughts are not true connections but the illness of OCD and the solution is to ignore the ringing telephone and not answer – or metaphorically put down the phone, so hanging up on those crossed lines and attributing them to a wrong connection. They are not valid messages, only jumbled up thoughts caused by an anxious state and transmitted by a tired brain that is overloaded and cannot cope. If one pays attention to anything so minutely and intently as an OCD sufferer does to his or her false messages, it is not at all surprising that this results in obsession.

Anxiety plus obsession and compulsion

The fact that OCD is a combination of anxiety, obsession and compulsion means that it can often be a very severe handicap. Like someone forced into hiding by death threats, people with OCD can find themselves virtual prisoners in their own homes, unable to go out of the door. Others with a less severe form of the condition find that a great chunk of ordinary life is closed to them. Not surprisingly, 'normal' people find this very hard to understand. They tend to think people with OCD are being silly or weak. What they don't understand is, that though the fears are unreasonable, the feelings they produce are every bit as real as those of someone who is being attacked by, say, a tiger. And that is not something that anyone would relish.

How rituals or compulsions are born

Anxiety levels rise in line with the amount of fear created by the way we think, and how we react to those thoughts. So, to begin recovery we must deal with the symptoms of anxiety, and start by taking charge of our physical reactions to panic and fear and to what we see as a 'threat'. Once we understand our bodily reactions, then we can tackle the thoughts and the values we place on them.

For example, I remember the first time I had to speak in front of a big audience. I was so anxious that my sight went blurred and my hearing all fuzzy. My heart was beating like a kettle drum and my left leg wouldn't stop wobbling. (You should recognize these as typical symptoms of fear.) It was a nasty experience, but I had to keep going. Once it was all over, I felt fine – my anxiety subsided and I felt relieved and confident. And, something miraculous happened, the next time I had to speak publicly, I wasn't so nervous and it was much easier to cope. Today, I can do it without much trouble, though I still feel a bit tense and anxious beforehand.

So once I had experienced the 'threat' and survived it, I became less and less sensitive to it. This is what happens to the majority of people in hundreds of different anxiety-making situations. By facing the 'threat' they learn that in practice it isn't all that serious, and that they can cope with it. Psychologists call this process 'conditioning'.

People with OCD travel a different path and so 'learn' exactly the opposite – when faced with the 'threat', they feel compelled to react to a certain urge or thought in a way which they think will reduce or eliminate the danger. As they react to the imagined threat (obsession) by doing a voluntary act (ritual or compulsion), their anxiety subsides – though it would have done anyway and this is important, as we shall see. They therefore 'learn' that the way to deal with anxious feelings is to carry out certain rituals which temporarily lower their anxiety. Unfortunately because they avoid the 'threat' they become more sensitive to it and more and more frightened of what will happen if they do not complete their ritual. In practice, what they actually are afraid of are the unpleasant thoughts and fear associated with some dire happening which they imagine will occur if they do not respond to their urge.

We can liken rituals (or compulsions) to the common practices used by most people to ward off ill luck. Knocking on wood, not walking under ladders, etc. – solutions which are supposed to keep us safe from simple superstitions. If you can equate OCD with hugely magnified superstition it becomes easier to comprehend.

So, what really is OCD?

As the name suggests, OCD usually means that the affected person suffers from obsessions and compulsions. Less frequently, the person may experience one but not the other. Obsessions are intrusive unwanted thoughts, ideas, urges, impulses or worries that repeatedly run through a person's mind. Almost by definition these will be alarming and repugnant. They may include:

- vivid images of killing or in some way abusing a loved family member;
- worries about dirt, germs, infection or contamination (affecting the person him or herself or family members);
- recurrent fears that certain activities have not been completed properly (even after countless repetitions);
- a need for certain objects (or even people) to be in 'correct' positions or places before activities can be undertaken;
- blasphemous thoughts;
- a fear that important things may be lost unless extreme care is taken;
- a fear that harm has been caused accidentally (running somebody over or leaving harmful objects or substances around);
- repetitive counting;
- weird or frightening images.

Other fears, which are sometimes on the line between a phobia and an obsession, might concern worries about the shape, functioning or smell of body parts.

As we have seen, compulsions/rituals are repeated behaviours that are usually performed to reduce the discomfort or anxiety generated by obsessive thoughts. These compulsions may include washing, checking, going back on journeys to see if someone has been harmed or sorting things into a 'correct' order. They are invariably excessive, usually having to be performed in a very precise manner and may be repeated many, many times until the person feels it is 'right'. Sometimes this behaviour does not seem to be directly related to relieving the obsession but those performing the ritual may still experience an overwhelming need to perform it.

Both obsessions and compulsions may vary greatly in duration and intensity among individuals. Depression can be a contributory factor, or may become a problem as a response to the level of handicap involved. As far as we can tell from recent research, in the UK at least 55,000 and possibly more are affected by OCD – some estimates say up to two million. The most common compulsions appear to be:

- excessive hand washing, bathing or showering;
- cleaning household equipment or furniture;

- avoiding 'contaminated' or 'dangerous' objects or substances (commonly dog faeces, knives, asbestos, etc.);
- checking water, electric and gas taps, windows, cupboards and doors;
- repeatedly checking that nothing 'bad' has happened or accidents have been caused, and demanding constant reassurance of this.

Less common ritual behaviours include:

- dressing oneself or children in a precise and predetermined fashion;
- entering or leaving the home or car in the 'correct' way, and repeating these behaviours.

Less common still are rituals concerning:

- hoarding, including an inability to throw things away without excessive checking or reading;
- performing certain acts (like dressing, bathing or crossing roads) very slowly.

Other types of OCD involve:

Controllability: We feel that we should be in control of our thoughts at all times. This is not possible. How could we premeditate every thought we have? So, people get very upset if they try not to think about something and it keeps coming back. Trying not to think of something actually encourages the thought to return and it increases the state of anxiety more and more. Also, constantly trying to think and reach for a solution can become part of the obsessive thought process.

Estimation of threat: Thinking that if this happens and that happens, then such and such will happen for sure. This train of thought is not exclusive to those with OCD.

Intolerance of uncertainty: Most of our lives we have to tolerate a bit of 'not knowing'. Not being 100 per cent sure. We can't guarantee everything so we have to endure patiently. We have to live with some degree of uncertainty.

Over-importance: Thinking that your thoughts may have some influence over a situation and that you have been or will be the cause of a disastrous outcome.

Responsibility: Feeling that you are very responsible for harm and its prevention.

Examples of obsessions	*Examples of compulsions*
Fear of shameful behaviour	Cleaning
Death and disaster	Washing
Contamination	Checking
Perverted sexual thoughts	Counting
Symmetrical arrangements	Measuring
Intrusive thoughts and images	Repeating actions or tasks
Lucky or unlucky thoughts	Hoarding things
Unsatisfactory body image	Confessing imaginary 'sins'

Why does someone become obsessive and compulsive?

Nobody can say for certain why any particular person develops OCD and there are several schools of thought. One is that abnormal functioning of the brain is mainly responsible. It is suggested that a chemical neurotransmitter or 'brain messenger' called serotonin is over-functioning, leading to extremes of social concern. The brain becomes overloaded with 'worry' messages, which spill into consciousness. Other clinicians relate OCD to 'hidden conflict' or early trauma, while some blame allergy, genetic predisposition (being born with a tendency towards it) or learning experiences during the early years. Of these, there is no evidence that allergy has an effect and most enquirers who have experienced only 'talking treatments' aimed at exposing psychological problems have reported little benefit.

   What we *do* know is that 'the stresses of life' can push someone into the downward spiral of OCD – divorce, separation, redundancy, bereavement or simply lousy living conditions and a run of bad luck. These things can depress and undermine the self-confidence of even the hardiest of individuals. Though, in a sense, it doesn't matter what the cause is and there is little to be gained by spending long hours agonizing about it and trying to root it out. We all have something in our background that could have triggered an OCD reaction – and no one's life is permanently happy and prosperous. Indeed, knowing the cause – even if it is the true one and not just a guess – isn't much help when it comes to treating the OCD. Whatever it was, you can't go back into the past and alter it. The problem is your badly conditioned behaviour and it is what you do in the future that will make a difference. Tackling OCD means learning to face – and overcome – the things that you fear. And that is precisely what this book aims to help you do.

10

The main OCD groups

The most common forms of OCD fall into clearly identifiable groups: obsessions and compulsive rituals; obsessions with counting rituals; obsessive thoughts without rituals; rituals without obsessive thoughts; slowness without visible rituals; decision-making difficulties.

Obsessions and compulsive rituals

Five main forms fall into this category:

- washing and cleaning;
- repeating sequences of actions;
- checking;
- orderliness and symmetry;
- hoarding.

Washing and cleaning

This is the most common problem reported to us at No Panic, where the person feels compelled to wash him or herself and almost everything he or she comes into contact with, usually in response to an obsessive thought pattern about the risk of contamination. The actual risk of harm to anyone through contamination in daily life is virtually nil. However, people with this form of OCD cannot convince themselves of this. They will often wash clothes, work-surfaces and themselves many times per day – even hundreds of times! They may use a variety of chemicals, such as bleaches and disinfectants, harming their own skin and ruining clothes.

Repeating sequences of actions

People with this form of OCD feel a compulsive urge to repeat a series of actions, often a specific number of times, before they feel it is safe to move on to the next task, whatever that may be. Equally they may well feel compelled to repeat tasks or rituals in order to ensure that harm does not befall anyone.

> **Tom** was in his mid twenties when his OCD started. He is not too sure what triggered it off, but it may have been linked to his superstitious nature. Whenever he went out he felt he had to touch certain lamp-posts in order to ensure that nothing awful happened to his mum and dad. But he found that as time went on, he had to touch more and more lamp-posts. He was having to leave the house for work earlier and earlier. By the time he sought help from his doctor, it was taking him two hours in the morning and two at night to get to and from work, whereas the actual journey time was about 15 minutes. His doctor got Tom to see a clinical psychologist. This therapist, using cognitive behaviour therapy (see Chapter 11), worked out a recovery programme with him. Tom, with a great deal of courage and hard work, began to tackle the problem. At the time of writing, Tom has reduced the time it takes him to get to and from work to half an hour each way and the number of lamp-posts that he has to touch is reducing significantly. He has managed to live with the anxiety it has caused him and, needless to say, nothing awful has happened to his mum and dad.

Checking

People with this form of OCD are obsessed with thoughts that something terrible, like a fire, will happen due to their negligence or carelessness.

> **Jane** had always been a carefree and happy-go-lucky person but, in her late twenties, things began to change. One day, when she went out she couldn't remember if she had switched the cooker off, so she went back to check. This kept on happening and the more she checked the more she felt she ought to go back and check again. The situation deteriorated rapidly until it was easier for her to stay at home than go out, so her outings became fewer and fewer. One of Jane's friends saw a No Panic poster in a Citizens' Advice Bureau and I'm pleased to say that with help and support, Jane is tackling her problem and is making a lot of progress.

There are other variations of 'checking':

- Some people are affected by the thought that they may have dropped something which might hurt someone. They will spend hours checking carpets, floors and chairs just to make sure everything is OK. They do not have any recollection of dropping anything but they cannot convince themselves of this without all the checking. It goes without saying that they rarely, if ever, find anything because they will almost certainly have been extra careful about not dropping things in the first place.

- Others are affected by the thought that they might have injured or killed someone. It is not unknown for people to continually scour their homes for traces of blood. Equally, car drivers in this group have been known to check their vehicle for damage every few hundred yards, and they will regularly ring hospitals and the police to check if there have been any accidents along their route. In many cases they have given up driving altogether as it is far less stressful.

Orderliness and symmetry

People with this type of OCD go far beyond what is 'tidy' to non-sufferers. It can involve many hours of checking and aligning, right down to fractions of a millimetre, to ensure that everything is just right.

Brenda's story began some 20 or 30 years ago. She noticed that she felt 'concerned' if things, like ornaments, weren't in exactly the right place or if the curtains weren't quite straight. Brenda tells it like this:

Nearly all of us like things neat and tidy and many people I know like things in a particular place or hanging in a certain place so I wasn't too worried at first. However, as time went on I began to feel more and more anxious if certain things weren't in *exactly* the right place – and I mean down to millimetres. Even my curtains had to hang in symmetrical lines. The only way to reduce my anxiety was to keep walking round and round the house just to make sure everything was as it should be. I would even wake up in the night, get up and sit looking at things just to make sure no one had moved anything. We even stopped having visitors in case they moved the cushions. I honestly believed I was going mad but I know now that OCD, like all anxiety disorders, has nothing to do with insanity. It is a nervous illness and not an illness of the brain.

I wish I had heard of organizations like 'No Panic' when I first became ill, because I don't think it would have got so bad if I had received help early on. But anyway by using cognitive behaviour therapy combined with an SSRI [selective serotonin reuptake inhibitor] anti-depressant I am 95 per cent recovered and haven't got much further to go.

A variation of this form of OCD is the office manager who cannot start work until all his pencils are sharpened to exactly the same length and are in exactly the right place. This exercise has been known to take him up to an hour and a half. Other examples are where things have to match exactly, for instance laces, and even eyebrows.

Hoarding

People with this form of OCD are unable to throw things away in case they may be needed at a later date or contain information which might be required at some time in the future.

In his late teens, **Roger** began to take a keen interest in the news and would read the newspaper from cover to cover, with the intention of being 'well informed', which was important to his job. If he couldn't finish the newspaper each morning, before he went to work, he would keep it to read in the evening. He wasn't particularly worried about this, even though sometimes it meant sitting up half the night, it was just part of the job. However, he began to feel a little unsure as to exactly what he had read so he started to hang on to old copies, just in case. Slowly but surely his bedroom began to fill up. He started to 'read' labels on cans and packets and to keep the labels just in case he had missed some important information. The rest of the story is all too plain: slowly his whole house filled up with newspapers, labels, tins and packets. He just couldn't bear to throw anything away, just in case.

Eventually Roger told his doctor about the problem and the anxiety it caused him. Although the doctor was not very familiar with OCD he did have some useful literature. Via this literature Roger got in touch with a local self-help group and with their support is following a programme of behaviour therapy and has recently started throwing a few things away. He knows it is a long, hard road but, having started, he feels confident that he can make a full recovery.

Other 'hoarders' include, for example, people who have to correctly identify pieces of music or quotes from books and therefore will hoard masses of paper on which are song titles, when they were a 'hit', and so on, and authors of books, when they were published, etc. As you can imagine, these 'lists' can, over a period of years, fill the whole house.

Obsessions with counting rituals

People with this form of OCD find that tasks or rituals have to be done a specific number of times or that some numbers are 'bad' numbers and if something adds up to a 'bad' number it has to be cancelled out.

Martin found that he had to do everything four times or in multiples of four. If he didn't do this he was obsessed with the thought that something awful might happen. If he was interrupted, he would have to start all over again. I am pleased to report that, with the correct support and knowledge, Martin is making a steady recovery.

Obsessive thoughts without rituals

People in this category find that their mind is continually engrossed in disturbing thoughts that are not relieved by any rituals. Examples would be: thoughts about harming themselves or others, thoughts about having carried out some evil or perverted deed, or thoughts of a blasphemous nature. There are a variety of ways of helping such sufferers, which include bringing the thoughts out into the open and getting them into perspective and/or the use of cognitive therapy to challenge the logicality of the thoughts and change the way the person thinks. Research shows that people with this form of the illness never actually carry out the deed with which they are obsessed.

Rituals without obsessive thoughts

This form of OCD, which is the rarest form, is where sufferers find themselves compelled to carry out strange rituals but not in response to any particular thought pattern. Once again behaviour therapy (see Chapter 11) holds the key to recovery, for example reducing the intricacies of the rituals or varying the times of day when they are done, or perhaps, when the ritual is about to be undertaken, encouraging a delay of five minutes and then of ten minutes, and so on. Learning to live with the anxiety this causes will, as in all anxiety disorders, slowly cause the anxiety level to progressively fall.

Slowness without visible rituals

This is a rare form of OCD and involves people whose behaviour is normal in most situations but who slip into a kind of slow motion when they tackle certain deeds or actions. The most common areas are taking a bath, getting dressed or crossing roads. These tasks may take an inordinate amount of time. Again, behaviour therapy techniques can help overcome this.

Decision-making difficulties

This tends to be found in combination with other forms of OCD. However, it can exist in its own right and it manifests itself in people with OCD taking an excessive amount of time to decide to do anything, such as deciding what to wear, where to travel, which can of food to buy. Once again it can be tackled using behaviour therapy.

11

Dealing with OCD

Distinguishing obsessions and compulsions

Many people fail to make a distinction between their obsessions and compulsions. It is easy enough to do when the compulsion is overt and behavioural, like washing the hands or checking the cooker to see if it is turned off. It's not so easy when someone feels compelled to engage in a mental act after having an obsessive thought. That mental act may be a prayer or something extremely personal that the person has to think about to counteract or neutralize the obsessive thought. It is important to keep in mind that, often, people are not aware of mental compulsions and it is imperative to make the distinction between the mental obsession and the mental compulsion. In therapy we talk about the desirability of accepting the obsessive thoughts, not trying to stop them, which is not really an option as it is impossible to stop a thought popping into one's head.

What we can do is tackle the compulsions, reducing them and ultimately ceasing to respond to the obsessions. This is the 'exposure and response' prevention principle. In some cases of OCD, the compulsion used by the person to negate a frightening thought is a mental process; in other words, first the 'obsessive thought' comes into the mind and then it is followed by the 'compulsive mental ritual'. Difficulties can occur when the covert or hidden ritual runs into the obsessive thought and the person has a problem in separating one from the other. It is very important that you are aware of this, so that the mental compulsion can be addressed.

Remember – OCD, like all anxiety disorders, can be overcome. You do not have to suffer the illness for the rest of your life.

So how do we deal with OCD?

Relaxation per se will not bring about a cure, but it is one of the pieces of the jigsaw we need to assemble to try to tackle OCD, so do take a look at the advice in Chapter 5. Another piece of the jigsaw is learning how to breathe from the diaphragm, evenly, smoothly and shallowly (see Chapter 4). This exercise alone will not bring about a cure either, but is of practical use when trying to cut down on compulsions.

Then the thoughts, a third section of the puzzle. How realistic are they? Is it likely that the horror being contemplated will actually occur? Will the action consuming every thought ever be carried out? A prospect that is dreaded? Here I hope I can give great comfort by stating categorically that the imagined nightmare will never happen. In fact, people who go through this kind of agony are usually extremely caring people, living in misery, and it is totally against their nature to cause harm. They are straining every bit of their minds and bodies to fight against the thoughts they are producing. Someone with OCD who is tormented by thoughts of harming is sickened by his/her ability to dismiss these thoughts and will never transfer thought into deed.

The media, television and newspapers, when reporting on cases of violent behaviour, use phrases like 'compulsively violent' or 'behaving obsessively', which is inexact. If we are going to use the term obsessive-compulsive behaviour correctly then we are talking about obsessions that upset people, not about deliberate thoughts and actions perpetrated by criminals. People with OCD are, as a group, usually gentle souls who don't get angry easily; in fact, they are often afraid of getting angry. Thinking that they might lose control is one of their worst nightmares. They may have grown up in a household where control and being proper is emphasized. They are often people with a strong sense of morality and being bombarded with unpleasant thoughts is unbearable to them.

Tackling obsessive thoughts

First, the goal is not to try and stop the obsessive thought – the more one tries to do that, the worse the problem becomes. There is no way that one can stop a thought coming into the mind. It's like hearing piped music in a lift or some public place and wishing you could switch it off but you can't. The sound is coming from beyond your reach. The goal is to be able to accept that the awful thoughts mean absolutely nothing and to be able to function with them present – to start learning to live with the noise, the thoughts, however loud they are playing, trying to do whatever you want to do, regardless of their insistence. As you progress, the thoughts will quieten, become less frequent and gradually fade away.

Standard forms of psychotherapy, focusing on trying to understand the meaning of the thoughts, are not only not useful but can be counter-productive. They mean that the therapist is taking your thoughts seriously. He or she is trying to find out how they fit into your character structure and it means too, that at some level, the therapist is viewing the thoughts as an indication of some genuine desire or tendency rather than recognizing them as alien and quite the reverse of your character. Therapy or counselling that concentrates on day-to-day issues or childhood problems, which the therapist thinks might relate to the content of your OCD, in most cases does not do anything to help either.

Another form of therapy, which is far more helpful, is cognitive behaviour therapy, Cognitive behaviour therapy (CBT) works on the OCD in two ways. First, cognitive therapy means helping the person with OCD to change the way he or she *thinks*, for example changing 'I need to wash 50 times' to 'I need to wash 45 times', etc., and challenging the thought that 50 washes are necessary by questioning the logic of the thought; for example 'If I needed to wash the plates 50 times wouldn't it say so on the label of the washing-up liquid bottle?' Second, behaviour therapy means changing the way the person with OCD actually *behaves* – so here perhaps helping to reduce the number of washes from 50 to 45 to 40 and so on, thus proving to the nervous system that a reduction is safe and that nothing awful will happen as a result of achieving the planned reduction.

CBT has a proven track record of success. It is only by slowly reducing the amount of things that you do, say or think, and by slowly facing the fears, that you will overcome the illness. (See Chapter 12 for details of self-help for OCD using cognitive behaviour therapy.)

How to withdraw from obsessive thoughts and rituals

We must learn to call intrusive thoughts and urges exactly what they are – obsessive thoughts and compulsions. This way we develop the ability to see the difference between what is OCD and what is reality. When an unwanted, frightening thought comes into the head of someone with OCD that person must learn to accept and realize for him or herself that 'this is not me but OCD'. For example: 'I think I might harm someone' is an obsessive thought and has no basis in reality. It must be recognized as no more than an error in transmission from a tired, anxious and exhausted mind. If someone with the disorder feels the desperate urge to wash, 'put something right' or check something, he or she must recognize this as OCD. It is that which is urging the person to ritualize, and by succumbing to the compulsions the person won't in fact change or alter any situation.

Once OCD has pervaded the thought processes it becomes an established habit, a repetitive way of thinking and that is why it is so difficult to break free from the rituals, but taking the following steps will help. Bear in mind that you may well need someone to help you with some or all of these steps – see Chapter 13 for more on how someone else can help.

- Allow the thoughts to come, and work or play regardless of them, accepting them as you would any background noise. An ignored thought that you place no credence on, gradually withers and dies from lack of nourishment.
- Don't encourage the thoughts to grow, flourish and even mutate. Give them nothing to feed on.
- Breathe from the diaphragm.
- Consciously relax all the muscle groups in the body.
- Put time between the thought and the compulsive behaviour. Start off with a very short period of time, a minute or two, even 30 seconds if the pressure is unbearable, and then allow the action to take place. During the pause, use the breathing technique, inhaling and exhaling slowly and evenly, relaxing your muscles as best you can, to help bring down the anxiety level.
- Lengthen this time space gradually until you feel that your anxiety level has dropped, and that you are more in control of your feelings and that, in fact, there is no point in ritualizing.

Nothing dreadful has happened and you have come through the crisis unscathed.

- Reduce the amount of actions you do to relieve anxiety. Reduction should be by a small amount, gradually decreasing the actions until they reach a stage that is an acceptable norm. Ask someone else (see Chapter 13, 'Getting help and support from others') to help you work out a programme to tackle this comfortably.

- Write a list of distractions to help postpone compulsive actions – perhaps something of a physical nature that will help to dissipate and reduce the level of anxiety. By this I mean some activity like walking briskly or running around the park, cleaning windows, digging in the garden, turning out drawers and cupboards, cycling, or maybe even dancing – in fact dancing is excellent, not only physically beneficial but mentally exhilarating, helping to lift the spirits.

This may all seem quite daunting and by now you may be feeling rather overwhelmed by the thought of having to follow all these suggestions. Don't worry – there's more detailed advice in the next chapter (Chapter 12, 'Self-help for OCD') on how to start breaking the problem down into manageable chunks, and how to tackle it at your own pace.

Imagined exposure

As we will see further in Chapter 12, exposure therapy can be very useful for tackling OCD – the aim being to actually stay in a feared situation until anxiety diminishes. If, however, someone engages in compulsive rituals because he or she fears some catastrophic event that can't be recreated – perhaps the country being swamped due to rising sea levels – then actual exposure must be replaced by imagined exposure. The person would explore the scene in detail as he or she sees it in the imagination, being encouraged to talk through feelings such as at what point in the scenario anxiety starts to rise, how likely it is to happen, whether it is connected with something seen or heard when going through a stressful time; imagining the event and enduring the anxiety and panic until it subsides.

If however you feel at a particularly vulnerable stage, you may be unable to cope with deliberately thinking of your worst nightmare, in which case, perhaps writing about some lesser degree of your anxiety to start with may be preferable. Try listing the problems in order of the amount of anxiety they cause, starting with something that causes the least amount of anxiety. Imagined exposure is like any other anxiety disorder therapy in the sense that it is good practice to create a hierarchy, a ladder, which starts with a lower intensity of anxiety and gradually increases the stages of exposure step by step.

Another method that suits some people is to put their story, including their fears, on tape and go through it over and over again, say for a minimum of an hour a day. You could split your listening into two half hours if you found an hour was too difficult to fit in with your lifestyle. This method will have an effect called habituation. The 'autonomic responsiveness' – the emotional reaction to the stimulus – will gradually diminish. If you watched a violent section of a play on videotape over and over again, it would slowly, by degrees, lose its emotional impact on you. You would find your mind wandering, perhaps noticing that the action wasn't very good and that the pool of blood on the carpet looked unreal, too much like tomato sauce.

The only danger with any of the exposure methods of recovery is that doing them intermittently, or just when you feel like it, will not work – practice, practice and practice again is the way to take charge of OCD.

Involving family members

Family members nearly always become involved with the OCD, so it is important that they understand what is going on and that they don't contribute to the disorder by giving inappropriate reassurance. People with OCD are constantly looking for someone to reassure them that all is well or to help them with their rituals. By this I mean helping them to complete their rituals, checking with them, bending to the pressure that the person with OCD can put on them through emotional blackmail. I don't think that emotional blackmail is too strong a phrase as it explains the desperate lengths someone with OCD will adopt to stem and quieten his or her internal turmoil. The more reassurance that is given, the more will be needed, until the family members are also drawn into and trapped by the illness.

So, family members must become skilled at knowing when it is right to be supportive and encouraging. Someone who is trying to stop ritualizing will appreciate that. In some instances it is beneficial to include family members and give them information that will help them understand OCD. How else can someone with no experience of OCD understand how anxiety can produce such extraordinary reactions? What spouses and family members can do is give praise when progress is made and maintained, encourage positive thinking, help change a professed negative outlook and so revive self-esteem. A goal that someone with OCD may achieve will probably seem to the uninitiated as small, even pathetic, but they must remember that to the person with OCD it will feel as if he or she has climbed a very high mountain. There's more on how to help in Chapter 13, 'Getting help and support from others'.

- *To those with OCD*: Cultivate a positive outlook. Look beyond the cloud of despair.
- *To family and friends*: Don't allow negative thinking. It will only produce misery.
- *To everyone involved*: Make an effort to be pro-active. You will reap the reward of reclaiming a calm, happy family member.

The search for a cure

People with OCD and other severe anxiety conditions are often desperate for a cure, but they are frequently disappointed. The fact is that no 'miracle cure' exists. There are no magic pills or potions you can take. Doctors can help, but they cannot cure. Drug treatment on its own seldom produces more than a temporary calming and may result in drug dependence.

Many people will try any new idea on offer – hypnosis, special diets and all sorts of other 'alternative therapies'. Though these are often expensive, very few people find them satisfactory. Therapy from an NHS psychologist or psychiatrist is much more likely to work – but unfortunately, these professionals are greatly overloaded and only have time to help a small proportion of the thousands of anxiety patients. The stark fact is that most people with OCD get no help or treatment at all.

However, as the following chapter shows, there is one treatment option that is widely available – self-help using cognitive behaviour therapy. This method involves changing the way you think combined with, where appropriate, a structured programme of facing up to the physical rituals and tasks in manageable stages, thus building up self-confidence and self-esteem. It is not a particularly quick method but it does offer long term benefits and many people have overcome their distressing symptoms using this approach.

12

Self-help for OCD

Self-treatment – exposure and changes to thinking patterns

Earlier I explained that most people learn to cope with anxiety by facing up to the things that make them anxious, thus making themselves less sensitive to fear. However, people with OCD somehow take a wrong turning and learn that anxiety goes away if they perform a certain action in a special way. Often the anxiety only goes away for a short time, though, and this produces further anxiety and the need to respond to the compulsion more and more.

Self-treatment gets you to do exactly what 'normal' people do – face up to your anxieties, your compulsions. This means deliberately exposing yourself to situations that make you feel anxious, until you become less sensitive. Cognitive-behavioural treatment encourages such self-exposure and will definitely cause you some uncomfortable moments, but you are going to undertake a training programme so that you can get there in easy stages, through a similar process to that outlined in Chapter 8.

Getting started

Before starting, look again at the 'Self-check' questions on page 55 to remind yourself of some basic facts. Talk to your GP about what you are planning to do and ask for specific guidance if you are on medication. If you are taking sleeping medicines and/or over-the-counter preparations such as St John's Wort, etc., ask his or her opinion about these. *Please tell your doctor what you are taking so that the GP can help you with your recovery.*

Most important of all, you need to work out exactly what makes you anxious – so first: write down on a sheet of paper *broadly* what you consider your OCD problem to be; second: note down all the unwanted, persistent, recurrent impulses, thoughts and/or images that make you feel most anxious.

Getting below the surface

I suggested you wrote a broad description of your OCD. Here is an example to show you what I mean.

> **Mary's** problem started in her twenties when she became obsessed with contamination, especially with dust and germs from dustcarts. It soon grew to include anything that may have been near a refuse tip, even a vehicle that may have driven by. Very rapidly, Mary became a prisoner in her own home, terrified to venture out in case she got contaminated by a passing car or something that may have fallen from it. On the occasions when she was forced to go outside, she would shower 300 times on her return. New clothes, which were delivered by mail order, had to be washed 100 times before she could wear them.

The above description of OCD has included the way in which Mary was affected by her illness in detail. Has your description included all the things that worry you and what you do to alleviate your anxiety?

Your second list should be a really accurate statement of what exactly makes you anxious. You might well list things like:

- being afraid of contamination in public lavatories;
- being afraid of swearing out loud in church;
- being afraid of stepping in dog faeces;
- being afraid of forgetting to lock the door, turn off the electricity, gas and/or water;
- being afraid of harming someone.

The next stage is to work out what it is about these situations that causes you a problem. For example:

- What kind of germs do you expect to be contaminated by in a public lavatory? What are the chances of you being contaminated? How many people do you think this happens to on average?
- What do you think might happen if you swore in church? Would you expect a disaster? Would you feel humiliated?

- What would happen to you if you stepped into some dog faeces? Would you become ill? Would your family become ill? What would happen?
- What would happen if you forgot to lock the door, turn off the electricity, gas and/or water? Would you be burgled? Would there be a fire, an explosion? Would your home be devastated? Would your family/friends be hurt?
- Why are you afraid of harming someone? Do you want to do this? Are you terrified of doing this?

Look back to where I asked you to write down what you considered your problem to be, in broad terms. Now think about it again in the light of what I have just been saying. What *really* frightens you in the situations you listed? Note down your considered version under two headings: 'These are the situations that make me anxious' and 'These are the things that *really* make me anxious in those situations'.

Obviously, it is important to be as accurate and truthful as possible. The most important part of self-exposure – which is yet to come – may not work properly if you don't get these issues straight at this stage.

Planning self-exposure and setting goals

You need to carefully plan your self-exposure programme, choosing specific goals, not vague ones and deciding what specific steps you need to take to reach them. Chapter 13 will show how family and friends can act as helpers.

Choosing specific goals

Your goals will be your objectives – the targets you want to achieve; and everyone's goals will be different. Here are some examples:

- 'I want to be able to leave the house without checking the door so many times.'
- 'I want to be able to walk the kids to school without panicking in case they tread in some dog dirt.'
- 'I want to be able to go to church and be calm.'
- 'I want to be able to go to a shop and try on new clothes.'

- 'I want to be able to go to bed without putting away all the kitchen knives.'
- 'I want to be able to go into public lavatories and only take the same precautions that "normal" people do.'

Notice that these goals are specific, that is, they talk about particular things the person wants to do. As we saw in Chapter 8, it is no good making vague statements like, 'I would like to live a normal life' or 'I want to feel better than I do at the moment'. The reason for being specific is that it is then much easier to plan your journey and much easier to tell whether you are getting there or not. In other words, specific goals let you measure your progress.

The goals you set should be related to the frightening situations that you listed previously – the precise things that frighten you. Thus in one of the examples I gave earlier, Mary, who was obsessive about cleanliness, might say: 'I want to be able to eat my meals with a knife and fork again, instead of having to use my fingers. I want to be able to touch things that other people have touched. I want to be able to do this without washing my hands so excessively.'

How many goals will you set yourself? Perhaps it will be five – but the number could easily be either smaller or greater. Do try to make sure that your goals are genuinely different ones, not versions of the same thing. Think about this carefully and then write down what your own personal goals will be. Make sure they are specific and that they cover the exact things that frighten you. It's very important that you get this right, because otherwise your self-exposure work may take you in the wrong direction.

The steps on the way

Right. You've set your goals, so you know what you are about to tackle. Now you need to list all the steps you are going to take to help you combat your OCD. These are the stages in your self-exposure programme, the steps on your journey to recovery.

Here is a typical example of the steps for Miss K:

Miss K. would really like to be able to go shopping in the town centre but it takes her so long to leave the house, she can't even get to the shop at the corner of her street. She has to keep checking and checking, again and again, the taps on her gas cooker. She checks them until she feels 'it's right' and moves into the next room but within minutes she is back in the kitchen checking again.

Working with a helper, she decided on five steps, each of which represented a more difficult task than the previous one. The steps broke the problem into manageable stages – she couldn't make the leap straight to the third step, because that was just too difficult for her. So the first two steps were included to help her get there.

There are several ways that Miss K. (and you) can help reduce checking. She might reduce the amount of times checked by an agreed and sensible amount, until an acceptable level is reached (writing down in the diary that the task had been completed). When anxiety begins to mount, some diaphragmatic breathing might help control the feelings being experienced. As each step is taken the level of anxiety should drop if the task is completed properly. This would take several steps to accomplish.

Another method might be for Miss K. to put time between the urge to check and the actual checking. The amount of time should be increased gradually until Miss K. comes to a point where the urge has died down of its own accord. In the beginning, waiting two minutes before checking can seem an eternity and using the breathing technique can again help with the symptoms of anxiety, but as the waiting time is lengthened and accepted it becomes easier. Eventually, the waiting time is so long that Miss K. feels that her crisis is over and it is unnecessary to check her gas taps after all.

Your steps need to be in the right order and this depends on how difficult the steps are. For example, a person with OCD may feel:

- fairly anxious about using a friend's lavatory;
- less anxious about going into the lavatory belonging to a member of the family;
- extremely frightened and anxious about using a public lavatory.

If this is so, then using the toilet belonging to the family member should come before using the friend's toilet and using the public toilet should come last.

How much anxiety?

As we saw in Chapter 8, self-exposure steps are all about facing up to anxiety and becoming less sensitized to the things that make you anxious: you do have to experience anxiety for this work.

But it is worth repeating that although your programme of steps represents a rising scale of difficulty, that does not mean you will feel more and more anxious as you go on. On the contrary: right now you may feel that Step 5 is going to be a lot more difficult than Step 1, but once you've dealt with Step 1 you will have already reduced your *total* level of anxiety, and Step 2 won't seem so bad. The same will apply as you move from Step 2 to Step 3.

Also, you are not being asked to face more anxiety than you can stand. All the research on this subject shows that though you do have to experience some anxiety, you don't have to experience a vast amount. A moderate amount of anxiety will do the trick and that is the whole point of doing things by easy stages.

A summary of the rules

Before you decide on the steps for your personal 'journey', here is a summary of the rules:

Rule one: Imagine a high wall made of bricks that you want to lower so that you can see over the top. As you reduce your rituals you are removing some of the bricks but be warned, take off too many bricks at once and your wall will collapse.

Rule two: Each time you remove some of the bricks remember that you must do it systematically, so keeping the wall intact and balanced. However, if you start to remove the bricks only one at a time, this might not raise your level of anxiety and won't get you anywhere. You must remove sufficient bricks to make you feel a little uneasy but not so many that you feel as if your wall is going to fall down.

Rule three: Remove as many bricks as you need to reach your goal. Some walls are higher than others and, if you are very frightened, the bricks may need to be removed more slowly. This is fine as long as you do not start to build up your wall again by reverting to previously reduced rituals.

Rule four: Steps taken to reach your goal can be measured in time as well. A step can be something like staying in a situation that makes you anxious for an agreed amount of time, then increasing that amount of time as you become more confident, building up the time lapse between the urge and the neutralizing action. Eventually, you will become bored with having to wait so long before you are allowed to check, count or whatever, and, as your adrenaline drops, you will begin to realize that it really isn't necessary to do your ritual. Nothing has happened and nothing ever will.

Rule five: Remember that every step is a valuable achievement in itself.

Your steps to your goals

You should now be ready to draw up your list of steps to reach your goals. Think carefully about the examples I have given and the five rules. Now start with the first goal on your list. Write it down as 'Goal No. 1' and write down a list of steps you will take to achieve that goal (use as many steps as you believe you will need): 'Step 1', 'Step 2', and so on. You will need to draw up a list like this for all the separate goals you intend to tackle and all the steps you need to take to reach these goals.

Now all you have to do is work your way through them – but before you begin, what about getting some help? The next chapter looks at how to use support from others so that the support helps but doesn't feed your problem.

13

Getting help and support from others

Helpers are people who will give you support as you carry out your self-exposure programme to tackle fears, phobias and OCD. They won't do anything to force you and they won't be there to tell you what to do – but it helps to know that they are nearby when you enter an anxiety-raising situation and that you have got someone you can talk to.

Helpers are also a 'crutch' to get you past exposure steps that are otherwise too difficult. They must not become a permanent fixture: the agoraphobics who say they are recovered because they can go anywhere – providing someone holds their hand – haven't recovered fully. Improved certainly: but the goal is always to be able to do things for yourself, the way that people who do not have phobias do.

In the same way, if you have OCD, helpers must again not become a permanent fixture and you must be careful not to involve them in your rituals. Asking constantly for reassurance will not be beneficial and will hamper your progress. Therefore, limit the amount of times you ask and reduce the reassurance in the same way as you are reducing your rituals. The goal is always to be able to do things for yourself, that way you will raise your self-esteem and have confidence in your ability to go forward towards recovery.

Your helpers may be people who have recovered from OCD or phobias and who now work as volunteers; friends; or family members. Volunteers are not all that numerous, unfortunately, so most people with anxiety disorders find that they have to rely on family and friends – and this is fine, provided that they go about it the right way. A family member or a close friend can be a great help to you, even if he or she finds it hard to understand the way you feel (we never really feel other people's pain the way they feel it themselves). You may find that others have all sorts of false ideas about OCD, panic, phobias (and about you), so it would be a good idea to get them to read through this book, or to contact a self-help organization such as No Panic for more information.

The messages that should get across to your helpers are these:

- 'People with phobias or OCD have not deliberately handicapped themselves and if we could "pull ourselves together", "snap out of it" or "stop being so silly", we would.'
- 'The feelings that severe anxiety gives us are an automatic body response and logical explanations are not the way to get rid of them: anxiety and phobias go much deeper than that.'
- 'There is no point in helpers getting angry or frustrated with a phobic person, or one who has OCD: it will only make recovery harder.'
- 'What family and friends should do is help us face the phobia or OCD through our self-exposure programme, rather than trying to talk or bully us out of it (even with the best of intentions).'

Discuss these messages with your helper (or helpers – there is nothing wrong with having several) to get your relationship going.

Preparing to help

Once you have settled on a main helper, it is important that he or she understands what you are trying to do. Make sure that your helper:

- reads this book through to gain an understanding of phobias, anxiety and OCD;
- understands what self-treatment is and how it works;
- knows what your goals are and why you have chosen them;
- know what your steps are and why you have chosen them.

Doing the quiz below should help you both.

Phobias/OCD – a simple quiz for you and your helpers

You should do this quiz first and then get your helper to do it. There are four possible answers to each question. Write down the one that you think is right. Check your answers on page 102.

Question 1. A phobia/OCD is:
(a) A mild kind of mental health problem.
(b) A disease.
(c) A set of deeply ingrained thoughts and habits.
(d) A personality weakness.

Question 2. Anxiety and fear are:
(a) Natural reactions which are often useful.
(b) A useless hangover from the days when people lived in caves.
(c) A sign of weakness or cowardice.
(d) Something we would be better off without.

Question 3. People are said to have a phobia/OCD when:
(a) They worry a lot.
(b) They experience strong feelings of fear in situations that don't pose a real threat.
(c) They experience feelings of fear when they are in danger.
(d) They feel frightened all the time.

Question 4. The symptoms of fear are actually produced by:
(a) Unpleasant thoughts going round and round in the mind which can increase fear.
(b) The pulse rate continually racing.
(c) Adrenaline released into the bloodstream inappropriately.
(d) Picking up 'bad vibes' from others, which can make people fearful.

Question 5. Phobias/OCD are made worse by:
(a) Staying in the situation that makes you anxious.
(b) Not having an easy 'escape route' when anxiety starts to rise.
(c) Reading too much about them.
(d) Avoiding the situation that makes you anxious.

Question 6. Finding out the root cause of someone's phobia or OCD:

(a) Is an essential starting point for recovery.

(b) Is useful for recovery but not essential.

(c) Is relatively easy to discover.

(d) Is not worth spending time and energy on.

Question 7. The commonest single type of phobia is:

(a) Fear of dogs.

(b) Agoraphobia.

(c) School phobia.

(d) Dentist phobia.

Question 8. The most effective way to overcome OCD/phobias is usually:

(a) By self-exposure treatment.

(b) With tranquillizers.

(c) By going into a psychiatric hospital for a period.

(d) By avoiding things that trigger it.

Question 9. The goals for recovery should be:

(a) Set as high as possible.

(b) Set at a realistic level.

(c) Set by a professional therapist.

(d) Set as low as possible.

Question 10. The steps towards the recovery goal should be:

(a) As close together as possible.

(b) Limited to five.

(c) Big enough to be worthwhile, but not so big as to be too difficult.

(d) As far apart as possible.

If either you or your helper got a lot of these questions wrong you really *must* go back and re-read previous chapters in this book. You are bound to run into problems if you start self-exposure with a lot of mistaken ideas.

A contract with your helper

Ideally, you should try to make a contract with your helper – an agreement that you will both stick to over the next few weeks. In many cases a verbal contract is sufficient; however, some people find that putting things into writing enables them to work more methodically.

The following is a suggested contract that you could draw up with your helper. You will both need to read it through carefully and sign it when you are both happy with everything in it.

Sample contract

CONTRACT BETWEEN:

_____ and

(your name)

_____

(helper's name)

I_____(your name)

declare that I am entirely serious in wanting to overcome my phobia/OCD and I promise to do my very best to carry out the programme of self-exposure work, which I have outlined for myself, taking the rough with the smooth and the failures as well as the successes, until I reach my goals.

I_____(helper's name)

declare that I understand the tasks that you are undertaking and the ways in which I can help. I promise to do my very best to help you carry out your self-exposure programme, taking the rough with the smooth and the failures as well as the successes, until you have achieved your goals.

SIGNED_____(your signature)

SIGNED_____(your helper's signature)

DATE_____

TO HELPERS

The rest of this chapter is for people who want to help someone with panic, phobias or OCD.

People with anxiety disorders will often get others, usually family members, to constantly reassure them that everything will be OK. In this way there is continual pressure on other members of the family to become part of the imagined solution to the problem. So, instead of learning to overcome their anxiety and fear, those with anxiety disorders have learned that certain 'happenings' will reduce the distressing feelings. They are then on a downward, slippery slope of thinking and doing more and more things so as to make life bearable, until they reach a point where their whole life is taken up with actions or thoughts which actually make 'normal' life totally impossible. It is important that a helper does not become simply another 'happening' in this process.

Can't people with OCD just pull themselves together?

No. If they could they undoubtedly would. OCD is not a straightforward condition like being pregnant, where either you are or you are not. The waxing and waning content, sometimes coupled to extreme pressures or rewards in daily life, can make it look as if the person is 'only as bad as they want to be'. This is invariably a false perception. Most of us are capable of supreme effort when the situation demands it, but cannot be expected to maintain this in everyday life.

Many people have vaguely obsessive habits of some sort. Some time ago I was talking to a group of young mothers (members of a social group, not women with anxiety disorders) and the conversation came round to cleanliness and then to lavatory rituals. They all had what might be described as irrational habits concerning using their own or other people's lavatories. These ranged from mild anxiety about infection that involved regular use of strong cleaning agents, to extreme anxiety requiring lengthy rituals (undressing, several washes or showering). None could be described as having OCD, but all were going beyond a reasonable level of care. All of them were relieved to find that they were not alone in their 'odd' behaviour. Other situations encountered have included people who use slight obsessions about 'correctness' to make them better at their jobs and those who put things in order as a calming precursor to a major activity. These are personality traits rather than symptoms of an illness and, as far as OCD is concerned, might be compared to the relationship between social drinking and alcoholism. The problem is that those of us who find slight obsessive behaviour rather useful often find it difficult to relate to people whose lives are dominated by obsessions.

Twelve handy tips for helpers

The hints and advice below come from many years of experience.

1 Find out as much as you can about OCD self-treatment but don't make out to be the expert. Only the person with the problem can solve it – your job is to assist in a friendly but not domineering way.

2 Don't try to talk someone out of their OCD – it doesn't work. Only experience and practice at self-exposure will change the person's behaviour.

3 Forget the fact that OCD is illogical. You have to remember that the fear is very real even if the thing that triggers it is harmless.

4 Try your best to understand the person you are helping but don't get emotionally involved in his or her progress.

5 The essence of being a helper is to maintain structured support – helping the person frame his or her programme and keep to regular planned activities with definite goals.

6 Don't threaten, nag, sneer or push too hard, that isn't help – it's just more pain. Once you have gained the person's trust you will know when a little pressure, joking or scolding will help.

7 Give praise and encouragement – these help build confidence and self-esteem.

8 The person with OCD must be in charge of the self-exposure programme, not the helper. Recovering from a severe anxiety condition means discovering that you are capable of controlling your own life.

9 Start reducing the level of support you give as soon as you can.

The OCD won't be beaten until the person can face it without you.

10 Be ready to take advantage of success – if an exposure step goes easily, suggest tackling the next one right away, while the going is good (but don't push this every time).

11 Accept that it won't always go smoothly – there will be hiccups, setbacks and sticking points, but 'two steps forward, one step back' is still progress.

12 Don't underestimate the weight of pain and fear an OCD person is carrying. People with the disorder, whose lives have been one long saga of defeat and discouragement, whose experience of the real world is that terrible things do happen to you, often feel pathetic and doomed to failure or ridicule, and find it difficult to have trust. They have all this to recover from as well as their OCD.

Panic – how to help

Dealing with panic that occurs as part of a phobia is relatively simple in that the panic will rapidly subside as soon as the person with the phobia escapes from his or her 'trigger' situation.

Dealing with a panic attack

A panic attack can be frightening to witness, and difficult to deal with, but the main area where you can help is by encouraging the person to regulate his or her breathing. Breathing in carbon dioxide will help to alleviate the attack – encourage the person to breathe in and out through cupped hands.

More long-term ways to help:

- Help the person use deep muscular relaxation, following the steps outlined in Chapter 5.
- Ensure a good diet is followed (see Chapter 6).
- Help the person identify and reduce unnecessary stress in his or her lifestyle.

Dealing with spontaneous panic is more difficult in that it happens suddenly without warning and is not necessarily related to a place or situation. Therefore you can help by noting when and where the panic happens. If a pattern can be established, then it will most probably turn out actually to be a phobic problem and should be treated as such, that is, using cognitive behaviour therapy.

One of the worst enemies of those who suffer from panic attacks is having nothing to occupy them when a panic attack happens. So, you can help the person to work out a 'panic plan', or list of things to do when an attack starts, such as jigsaws, tapestry, painting. The aim is to find activities which can be done without too much stress, which will stop the person sitting there feeling sorry for him or herself – a situation likely to cause the panic to escalate and take longer to go away. A good idea is to encourage the person to take a brisk walk or engage in other physical activity (see p. 38), which will burn off the surplus adrenaline and so help the panic to subside.

There are other ways in which you can help:

- Simply being there and showing you care goes a long way.
- Stay calm and don't ask questions at the time of the panic. Questions can be left until the panic has passed.
- Do not over-react with comments like 'Shall I get an ambulance or the doctor?' The person is already terrified, so please avoid creating more panic. The person knows, deep down, that the panic always passes.
- Try to get the person to breathe slowly. Rapid breathing stimulates the panic – the person needs less oxygen, not more.
- Don't make fun of the person during a panic attack. Gentle soothing comments will be of much more help.
- Remind the person to try and carry out deep relaxation. This is often difficult during a panic attack but getting the person into a relaxed position will help.
- Give the person all the love, care and support you can.
- Make sure the person carries out regular deep relaxation, it needs to become a daily habit and will help to prevent panic attacks occurring in the future.

- Hang on in there, it may be a long hard road to recovery but it will be worth it.

The latest research available indicates that one in three, or about 20 million people in the UK will experience a panic attack at some stage during their lifetime. So, you can see that it is a major health problem and needs to be dealt with like any other illness.

Phobias – how to help

Phobias affect millions of people in the UK, and the extent to which they are affected varies enormously. To take just one example, at No Panic we have one member who can fly around the world with her husband and yet cannot walk to the end of her road on her own. One of the most frustrating things for others is not being able to understand why on one day a person can do a particular thing yet finds it very hard if not impossible to do it the next. The person probably does not understand it him or herself and thus finds it very hard to explain. Most people get up in the morning feeling different from the previous day, so perhaps it is just about the way we feel when we start the day, or perhaps we haven't slept well and so, unknowingly, we are more tense on some mornings than on others. Deep relaxation, practised first thing in a morning, will certainly help to overcome this problem.

There are several ways you can help a person with a phobia:

- Be patient.
- Never support or take part in new avoidance patterns (in phobias) or rituals (in OCD). It is easier to say no the first time than to stop them once they have started.
- Keep the person's stress and anxiety levels as low as possible. Stress makes phobias worse. If you feel the need to 'let off steam', try not to do it in front of the person.
- Be consistent in what you say and do. Make it perfectly clear what you will and won't do.
- If you want the person to do, or not do, something, give some advance warning. If you suddenly 'spring' something on the person, he or she will tend to go into a panic or might do so through feeling 'rushed'.

- Give the person as much encouragement as you can, it really will help.
- If the person is referred for treatment, make sure that he or she keeps the appointment and is open with the therapist. Also, ensure that the treatment is specific to phobias or to OCD and is not general psychiatric or psychological treatment, as otherwise it will not necessarily overcome the problem. It may just help the person to relax but this is only one part of the remedy.
- Try not to let the person take a break from working on his or her recovery programme because this will almost certainly be a step backwards. Be firm but not domineering.
- Don't accept excuses like 'I can't try today because I've got a cold' or 'I've got a pain in my leg'. Usually these are part of the 'avoidance' habit and should be firmly discouraged. After all, a cold never killed anyone.
- Don't lose interest if progress is slow. It is a tough task the person is taking on.
- Don't put too much pressure on as it will be resisted – usually by the person not trying at all. This is one of the most difficult aspects of the helper's role but can be achieved with practice. Coaxing not bullying works best.
- Give praise when even the smallest step forward is made. Often a little present or reward will give further encouragement and incentive.
- Don't make fun of the person's problem. It is a genuine illness and negative or sharp comments will do nothing to help him or her get better.
- Hang on in there – the person you're helping wants to get better just as much as you want him or her to.

In conclusion, it must be acknowledged that the role of a helper is an extremely difficult one, so please remember there are support groups for helpers and carers as well as for those with anxiety disorders (see Useful addresses on pages 112–14). Often, carers too are prisoners of the person's fear, but with your support, love and affection, the person can get better. Life does not always have to be 'fear' dominated.

Answers to the quiz questions on pages 93 and 94:

Question 1. (c) OCD/phobias are a set of deeply ingrained thoughts and habits.

Question 2. (a) Anxiety and fear are natural reactions, which are often useful.

Question 3. (b) People are said to have OCD/phobias when they experience strong feelings of fear in situations that don't pose a real threat.

Question 4. (c) The symptoms of fear are produced when adrenaline is released into the bloodstream inappropriately.

Question 5. (d) OCD/phobias are made worse by avoiding the situation that makes you anxious.

Question 6. (d) Finding out the root cause of someone's OCD is not usually worth spending time and energy on.

Question 7. (b) The commonest single type of phobia is agoraphobia.

Question 8. (a) The most effective way to overcome OCD/phobias is usually by self-exposure treatment.

Question 9. (b) The goals for a recovery programme should be set at a realistic level.

Question 10. (c) The steps towards the recovery goal should be big enough to be worthwhile but not so big as to be too difficult.

14

Coping techniques and final stages

I have continually stressed that you can't get better without feeling anxious, and you can't fight the fear without facing up to it. It is also true to say that facing the situation head on, without any concealment or pretence, is by far the best and quickest way to overcome the condition. You need to experience the fear as it was learnt, in all its unpleasantness. It is no good trying to deal with a watered-down version: this will still leave you unable to face the real thing. You can't recover fully until you experience your anxiety in its worst form, pass right through it and learn that it can't really hurt you.

By now you have a lot more going for you than when you started:

- You have a series of achievements behind you.
- You have built up your strength and self-confidence.
- You know you can do things that once you thought you couldn't.

Taking your mind off it

There are three ways of reducing tension:

- by distracting your mind;
- by concentrating hard;
- by doing something physical.

Give yourself a 'talking to'

The other obvious thing to do is to keep telling yourself encouraging things like:

- 'I'm going to try as hard as I can.'
- 'The worse I feel the better it's going to make me.'
- 'Sticks and stones can break my bones, but OCD fears can't hurt me.'

Perhaps you have already discovered some of these techniques for yourself, if so, make a note of them. If not, make a note of what appeals to you, as 'Technique 1, Technique 2', and so on.

Practising your coping techniques

You have now chosen some coping techniques, but you won't know for certain if they are going to help you until you have tried them out. Before you read on:

- During your next exposure session, try out your coping techniques and see how well they work.
- If they don't work for you, change them and try others until you find at least one that does.

You might also write down some encouraging thoughts:

'These are only feelings and I haven't died or gone mad or run off screaming.'
'These feelings do not mean I'm going to have a stroke or a brain haemorrhage.'
'This will only last so long then it will start to get better.'
'This is the ultimate horror – if I can handle this, I can handle anything.'

The final stages

As you approach the final stages of your recovery, you should:

- make a careful review of the progress you have made so far;
- decide how close you are to recovery;
- decide whether to press on with self-exposure.

How far have you come?

Think carefully about the statements listed below and choose the one which most closely resembles your situation:

1 I am completely cured of my OCD.
2 I am almost cured but there are still one or two situations that I avoid.

3 I can do much more than I used to, but I haven't actually reached any of my original goals.
4 I have made a little progress and I am still trying, but I get stuck easily.
5 I haven't made any progress worth mentioning and I can't keep up daily self-exposure practice.
6 I feel worse now than when I started.

Whichever statement you chose, you'll find some useful advice below. But before you read on, it's worth knowing that at this particular stage of a self-exposure course, even people who have made very good progress often feel fed-up, 'flat' and down, apprehensive about the future, and uncertain about the changes that may be on the way.

Let's face it, when you recover from OCD life is going to be very different. Sometimes, emerging from an anxiety disorder is like being freed after many years. Things have changed while you have been locked in your own personal prison. Life is full of new challenges and opportunities and it can be bewildering. It is a new world, but the main thing is that it is no longer a dangerous one. Try to be positive about the new world you are entering and don't let the fresh air and freedom get you down.

Now let's go back to the last questionnaire:

If you chose 1: Congratulations! But go back and recap because there may be some fears you have still not rooted out.

If you chose 2: Well done! But go back and recap because you still need to sort out the last remaining fears.

If you chose 3: Fine – you have achieved a lot! Go back and recap and keep up the regular practice.

If you chose 4: Don't worry, you'll get there – and every step forward is a valuable achievement! You've shown you can make progress, but perhaps you need longer to practise. Go back and recap, making sure that your understanding is correct.

If you chose 5: Don't worry – it may be that you weren't quite ready to tackle a tough series of challenges like this, but there is no reason why you cannot have another go at improving your situation. Take a step back, build your self-esteem and confidence; re-read the information for recovery. Figure out what went wrong with your first attempt and then pluck up your courage again and proceed.

If you chose 6: I'm sorry to hear that, but it doesn't mean you are a hopeless case – just that it didn't work out this time. You need to take your time and avoid forcing your way forward, this will only build up your anxiety level. Concentrate on desensitizing your mind and body through muscle relaxation and calm, shallow breathing. When you feel less stressed re-read the information for OCD recovery and try again, but take it slowly 'one-step-at-a-time'.

If you chose statement 5 or 6, it is probably because you felt like Mary.

> **Mary** was severely handicapped by OCD, she had tried all sorts of treatment and had never got very far. She had very little confidence in herself, and her family had become very frustrated with her. Basically, they had given up on her because they thought she simply wasn't willing to make the effort to recover. Mary spent all day sitting at home feeling miserable and helpless, while the others got on with their normal lives.
>
> She decided to make one last effort, and joined a self-help group. Unfortunately, when it was time to take part in the self-exposure 'working group', she found the sessions so terrifying and draining that after two or three she gave up and stopped going. 'It's no good – I'm just a failure,' she told her friend miserably. 'I'm fated – there's nothing I can do. Perhaps one day someone will find a cure.'

It's easy to feel a failure, especially if you start off with very little confidence or energy, and then have a series of misfortunes and setbacks. But never despair, because there is no such thing as a 'hopeless case', though of course there are definitely people who find recovery more difficult than others. Are any of these statements true of you:

(a) I was very unsure and not at all confident to begin with and didn't really believe I could do it.
(b) I have been very depressed in general.
(c) I need to take a lot of sedatives just to get through the day.

(d) After I started the course, something happened which lowered my spirits and that was when it all went wrong.

If you feel that any of these sum up your position, the message is: You can still do it if you try again, but you need to get that problem sorted out first. It's most likely that you simply identified with (a) – that is, you were at a very low ebb to begin with, and so had further to go and needed to do more work. An extra large workload is no joke, but that doesn't make it impossible. For example, you need to put in much more effort to dig over a whole field than you do to dig over a small back garden – but you *can* do it, even if it looks like a daunting task to begin with.

What it actually means is that:

You need more encouragement
You need more help and support
You need to take it in easier stages

What to do:

- Discuss your problems with your helper and/or, for example, the No Panic Helpline.
- Make contact with local self-help volunteers.
- Plan to re-read this book and try again.

A fair amount of progress

This section is for you if you chose statement **3** or **4**.

The main thing I would like to say is that you have done well – perhaps better than you think. It isn't easy to re-conquer whole areas of life that your OCD has stolen from you. Above all, you shouldn't feel despondent that you haven't reached all your goals. The things you have achieved are well worth having.

Check your diary, your 'Goals' and your 'Steps' towards your goals. Now write down the five most important things that you have succeeded in doing – things that you could not do before.

You see! Real achievements! You may have been a bit slower than you hoped and you may not have achieved perfection yet, but that is nothing to be worried about. All progress is useful but be aware, you can lose it if you don't keep working on your problem.

What to do

Don't rest on your laurels. Think about how you can continue to push your OCD back. You've proved you can do it – but perhaps you need:

- more help and support,
- more time,
- a more careful look at your 'sticking points'.

Nearly recovered

This is for those of you who chose statement **1**.

Have you really overcome your OCD? I don't want to doubt your word, but it is all too easy to indulge in a little self-deception. Unless you completely eradicate your fears, there is always a likelihood that one day they will return. That's why I have to ask whether you have *really* overcome your OCD. As long as you still fear it – it lives on, it's still a danger. If after reading this section you aren't entirely sure you've recovered fully, go on to read 'Well on the way to recovery?, below.

Well on the way to recovery?

This is for those of you who chose statement **2** or who chose **1** and have since had second thoughts. Think carefully about what remains to be done, consult your diary and your original 'Goals', then list the tasks you still have to undertake before you are completely free of your fears.

There's no question that you have achieved a great deal. You can do many things that were once impossible and perhaps you have got rid of some of your fears altogether. This is very good. But it is absolutely vital to keep moving forwards. Don't stop while there is still work to be done. Experience clearly shows that for a person recovering from OCD, there is no such thing as standing still. Either you make progress, or eventually you will slip back again and that would be a great shame. Not because it means you are a failure, but because you then have to do the work all over again.

So now is the time to make a sustained effort to reach your goals, and before you do this, it is a good idea to make a careful review of what remains to be done. (I know you've just listed the main remaining tasks, but it's important to do it systematically.)

- Look carefully at the tasks you listed. Do they still fit the goals you originally listed? If not, do you need to alter your goals, or your tasks, or both?
- If necessary, draw up a new list of goals and/or tasks.
- Think carefully about the things you have achieved so far. Have you really become completely confident with them?
- Keep practising exposure to these things, until you are so relaxed in those situations that you actually get bored.
- Think carefully about situations you still find frightening or impossible to handle. Make sure you identify *all* of them.
- Make certain that all the situations you fear – without exception – feature in your list of goals and tasks.
- Think carefully about the steps that lead up to your goals. If you have changed goals, or included new ones, have you worked out steps to match? You may need to write out new diary sheets for new goals and tasks.

At the advanced stage you have reached, it really is worth the extra effort needed to root out your fears completely, but to achieve this you will need to do three things:

1 If you still fear panic, then this must be dealt with. You need to experience the panic and cope with it.
2 Throw away your props and crutches.
3 Do without your helpers.

You need to be free from intrusive thoughts, free from the anxiety that they cause you and by doing it yourself, alone, of your own free will, you will finally rout out the fears which have held you down for so long.

Into the panic zone

As I have repeatedly said, you have to experience and face your most anxiety-provoking situations, thoughts and objects, to become really recovered. It follows that unless you are prepared to experience severe anxiety – and perhaps panic – in those situations you dread, you will never fully recover, because:

- By experiencing your maximum level of anxiety, your whole body learns that fear won't actually harm you.
- By deliberately relaxing, your whole body learns that panic symptoms soon go away.
- By repeating the experience, you will soon find it doesn't make you panic at all.

The only reason why certain things make you afraid is that you run away from them. Stick in there, and you will get better. Avoid and you will get worse.

If you find this prospect too much to cope with, go back to the earlier parts of the course and work through them again. If necessary, go back through the whole business of choosing, practising and designing mini-steps to take you through the most difficult situations, and so on.

But right now I am urging you to go one step further: you must experience your worst fears. All your exposure work up to now has been geared to make you fit and confident enough to do this, so it isn't the bogey it once was, but as long as you experience anxiety in your trigger situations you need to practise going through it. When, at last, you find that whatever you do you are no longer anxious, consider yourself virtually cured. It is the imaginary dangers that you need to overcome, not the real ones. Be careful though. You are allowed to avoid things that genuinely might cause you worry, because this is the rational thing to do – but you must make an honest assessment. Are you really taking a logical decision and 'rationalizing' your fear by telling yourself, 'I find this unpleasant for genuine reasons, so I am entitled not to do it?' Only you can answer that question, but it is a crucial one.

Plan for the future

Don't let up until you are fully recovered, and then take full advantage of the new freedom you have won. The world is a big place, so get out and about and enjoy yourself. There's no need to limit your social life in any way or stay in one work area. You can go anywhere now. You take your cure with you. You don't have to keep your personal relationships the way they were when you were a prisoner of fear. You're free now and if people around you have trouble coming to terms with this, that's their problem, not yours. Never allow anyone to try to keep you in your cell.

One important question is often asked at this stage by those recovering from OCD: 'Will I ever have OCD again?' The honest answer to this is that, yes, you might, because no one can predict the way your life will unfold, but:

- OCD is less likely now. It's running away from anxiety that makes a temporary fear into a long-term anxiety illness.
- If it does recur, it will be a coincidence, not because you are particularly prone to the condition.
- If it does recur, you will know how to get rid of it and, with all the practice you've had, it will be much easier the second time around.

Congratulations – if you have done nothing else but read this book you have demonstrated that you want to tackle and overcome your illness and have taken the first major step.

Useful addresses

Alcoholics Anonymous
PO Box 1
10 Toft Green
York YO1 7ND
Tel.: 0845 769 7555 (24 hours a
day, 7 days a week)
Website: www.alcoholics-
anonymous.org.uk

**Anxiety UK (formerly the
National Phobics Society)**
Zion Community Resource Centre
339 Stretford Road
Hulme
Manchester M25 4ZY
Helpline: 08444 775 774 (9.15 a.m.
to 9 p.m., Monday to Friday)
Website: www.anxietyuk.org.uk

For those with anxiety disorders,
this group publishes a range of
leaflets and videos, a quarterly
journal (*Anxious Times*), and CDs
and DVDs on relaxation.

**British Association for Applied
Nutrition and Nutritional
Therapy (BANT)**
27 Old Gloucester Street
London WC1N 3XX
Tel.: 08706 061284
Website: www.bant.org.uk

The Association provides a list of
nutritional therapists.

**British Association for
Behavioural and Cognitive
Psychotherapies (BABCP)**
Victoria Buildings
9–13 Silver Street
Bury BL9 0EU
Tel.: 0161 797 4484
Website: www.babcp.com

This organization provides online a
directory of psychotherapists.

**British Association for
Counselling and Psychotherapy
(BACP)**
BACP House
15 St John's Business Park
Lutterworth
Leicestershire LE17 4HB
Tel.: 01455 883300 (general
enquiries)
For finding a therapist: 0870 0443
5220
Website: www.bacp.co.uk

The Association provides a search
facility for therapists online.

**British Psychological Society
(BPS)**
St Andrew's House
48 Princess Road East
Leicester LE1 7DR
Tel.: 0116 254 9568
Website: www.bps.org.uk

The Society has a directory of
chartered psychologists, some
of which may practise cognitive
behavioural therapy.

Depression Alliance
212 Spitfire Studios
63–71 Collier Street
London N1 9BE
Tel.: 0845 123 2320
Website: www.depressionalliance.
org

Directgov
Website: www.direct.gov.uk

This is a portal to public service information from the UK government, including directories and news and information of relevance to specific groups. The health and well-being section provides advice on accessing NHS health services.

Eat Well, Be Well
Website: www.eatwell.gov.uk

This is the Government's Food Standards Agency, and it gives advice on healthy eating.

FearFighter (Computerized Cognitive Behaviour Therapy)
CCBT Ltd
Tudor Court
14 Edward Street
Birmingham B1 2RX
Tel.: 0121 233 2873
Website: www.fearfighter.com

A method for delivering cognitive behaviour therapy via the individual's own computer.

First Steps to Freedom
PO Box 476
Newquay
Cornwall TR7 1WQ
Tel.: 0845 120 2916 (helpline open 365 days a year: 10 a.m. to 10 p.m. Monday to Thursday; 10 a.m. to midnight Friday to Sunday)
Website: www.first-steps.org

Aimed at those with phobias, OCD, general anxiety, panic attacks, anorexia and bulimia.

Food and Mood Community Interest Company
PO Box 2737
Lewes
E. Sussex BN7 2GN
Website: www.foodandmood.org

The Company points to the link between diet and mental and emotional health, and provides dietary self-help resources to help improve them.

FRANK
Helpline: 0800 77 66 00 (24 hours a day, 7 days a week)
Website: www.talktofrank.com

Provides information about drugs and how to get help in confidence with drug problems.

GAIAM Direct
Tel.: 0870 241 5471
Website www.gaiamdirect

Mail-order supplier of a range of exercise DVDs and related fitness products.

Meditainment Ltd
Kingsway House
134/140 Church Road
Hove BN3 2DL
Tel.: 01273 325136
Website: www.meditainment.com

Supplies CDs and audio downloads with creative visualization exercises for relaxation, self-development and self-discovery.

Mind
15–19 Broadway
London E15 4 BQ
Mind*info*line: 0845 766 0163 (9
a.m. to 5 p.m., Monday to Friday)
Website: www.mind.org.uk

Provides information about all
aspects of mental health, including
details of your nearest Mind
Association

NHS Choices
Website: www.nhs.uk

An online resource of health
information, factsheets and
information of local health
services.

NHS Direct
Tel.: 0845 4647 (24 hours a day,
every day)
Website: www.nhsdirect.nhs.uk

The telephone helpline provides
health information and advice
from nurses. The website provides
health information and allows you
to search for local health services
(GPs, dentists, opticians and
pharmacies) in your area.

NO PANIC
93 Brands Farm Way
Telford
Shropshire TF3 2JQ
Tel.: 01952 590005
Helpline: 0808 808 0545
(freephone; staffed every day
10 a.m. to 10 p.m. by trained
volunteers; answerphone service 10
p.m. to 10 a.m.)
Website: www.nopanic.org.uk

This charity has a range of self-
help materials, and runs telephone
recovery groups which are specially
useful for agoraphobics.

Samaritans
Helpline: 08457 90 90 90
Also provides support via
correspondence: Chris, PO Box 90
90, Stirling FK8 2SA
Website: www.samaritans.org

SANE
First Floor, Cityside House
40 Adler Street
London E1 1EE
Saneline: 0845 767 8000 (helpline,
6 p.m. to 11 p.m. 365 days a year)

The helpline provides information
and crisis support.

Stop Smoking Service (NHS)
Helpline: 0800 022 4332
Website: www.gosmokefree.nhs.uk

As well as the helpline, local
support sessions are offered to help
people give up smoking.

Triumph Over Phobia (TOP UK)
PO Box 3760
Bath BA2 3WY
Tel.: 0845 600 9601
Website: www.triumphoverphobia.
com

A national network of structured
self-help groups for people with
OCD and phobias (including
agoraphobia) to overcome their
problems using self-exposure.

Further reading

Bourne, Edmund J., *The Anxiety & Phobia Workbook*, Oakland, CA: New Harbinger Publications, 2005

Butler, Gillian, *Overcoming Social Anxiety*, London: Robinson Publishing, 1999

Cheevers, Peter, *Coping with Family Stress*, London: Sheldon Press, 2007

Dryden, Windy, *Overcoming Anxiety*, London: Sheldon Press, 2000

Ingham, Christine, *Panic Attacks*, London: HarperCollins, 2000

Kennerley, Helen, *Overcoming Anxiety*, London: Robinson Publishing, 1997

Lader, Malcolm, *Tranquillizers and Antidepressants – When to Take Them, How to Stop*, London: Sheldon Press, 2008

Marks, Isaac M., *Living with Fear*, New York: McGraw-Hill Education, 2005

Rowe, Dorothy, *Beyond Fear*, London: HarperCollins, 2007

Searle, Ruth, *Overcoming Shyness and Social Anxiety*, London: Sheldon Press, 2008

Silove, Derrick and Vijaya Manicavasagar, *Overcoming Panic*, London: Robinson Publishing, 2007

Tallis, Frank, *Understanding Obsessions and Compulsions*, London: Sheldon Press, 1992

Trickett, Shirley, *Coping with Anxiety and Depression*, London: Sheldon Press, 1996

Weekes, Claire, *Essential Help for Your Nerves*, London: Thorsons, 2000

Williams, Chris, *Overcoming Anxiety: A Five Areas Approach*, London: Hodder Arnold, 2003

Index